THE RAIN BARREL EFFECT

THE RAIN BARREL EFFECT

HOW A 6,000 YEAR OLD ANSWER HOLDS THE SECRET TO FINALLY GETTING WELL, LOSING WEIGHT & FEELING ALIVE AGAIN!

Dr. Stephen Cabral

Copyright © 2017 Cabral Research LLC
All rights reserved.

ISBN-13: 9781975774837
ISBN-10: 1975774833
Library of Congress Control Number: 2017913602
CreateSpace Independent Publishing Platform
North Charleston, South Carolina

Standard Disclaimer

Legally we are required to share with you this standard disclaimer: Although the author and publisher have made every effort to ensure that the information in this book was correct at press time, the author and publisher do not assume and hereby disclaim any liability to any party for any loss, damage, or disruption caused by errors or omissions, whether such errors or omissions result from negligence, accident, or any other cause. The author and publisher also disclaim liability for any possible consequences or medical outcomes that may occur as a result of applying the methods suggested in this book.

The information contained in this book is the opinion of the author's and does not replace professional medical or nutritional advice. Dr. Stephen Cabral does not provide medical advice or engage in the practice of medicine. This book is provided for your general information only and is not intended as a substitute for the medical advice of physicians. It is intended to provide helpful knowledge and informative material on the subjects addressed in this publication. The reader should regularly consult a physician in matters relating to his/her health and particularly with respect to any symptoms that may require diagnosis or medical attention. All readers who are taking any form of prescription medication should consult with their physicians before making any changes to their current eating habits.

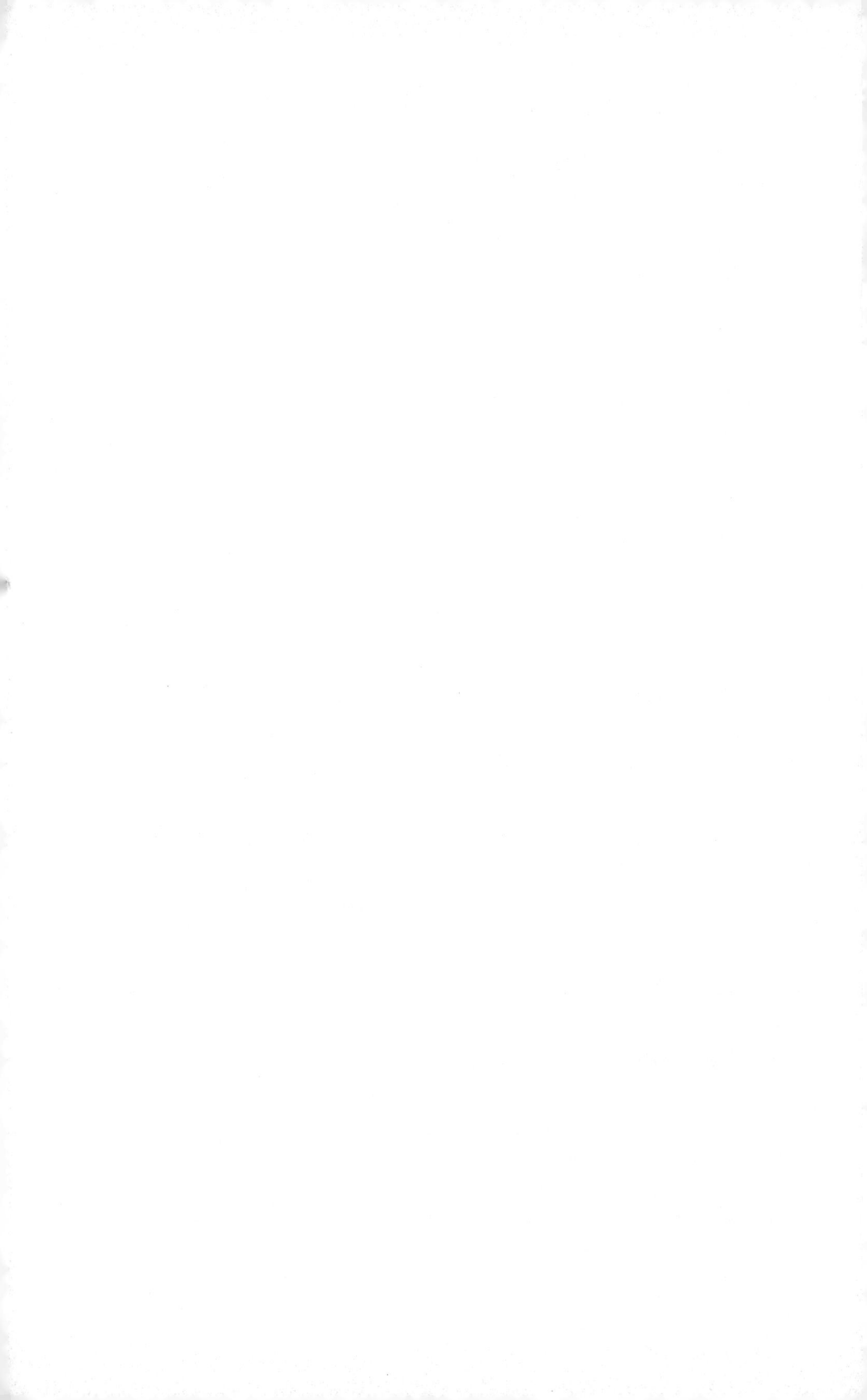

Dedication

To my parents,
for always letting me find my own path in life.

To my wife,
for believing in me since the beginning & supporting me
every step of the way.

To my 2 girls,
for helping me discover what life is all about.

100% of this book's profits are donated to charity

Thank You

Thank you to the thousands of people my team and I have been fortunate enough to work with. Below is a small sample of their success stories in their words:

15 YEARS OF DIGESTIVE ISSUES RESOLVED

"Dr. Cabral has as changed my life. For more than 15 years I have struggled with digestive issues and what many doctors have called IBS. I've had no success with traditional medicine and found their treatment (often antibiotics) to just make matters worse. I now remain symptom free and have become much more educated on nutrition/self care/and a balanced life style.

- Christine P.

VIRUSES ELIMINATED

"After getting the norovirus in 2006, it has taken me years to recover my health. I've seen numerous physicians & holistic health providers over the years, and Dr. Cabral has, by far, been the most helpful. He is a brilliant and skillful physician, and he will help you get to the bottom of any health issue, no matter how complex."

- A.J.

FINALLY... A FULL RECOVERY

"After years and years of symptoms following eating including gas, bloating, cramps, excessive burping, etc. I finally got REALLY sick with SIBO and couldn't eat anything at all. Was living on an elemental (predigested) formula and honestly had no hope anything would ever get better.

I saw 3 gastroenterologists, 2 PCP's, and multiple other physicians and healthcare providers and they all just kept recommending drug after drug (prilosec, etc. etc.) or inconclusive tests over and over. After almost 5 rounds of Xifaxan I had had enough. My friend had recently been cured by Dr. Cabral, so I decided to give it a shot. By the end of my first visit I knew I was in the right hands. I completely turned my entire care over to him and followed his recommendations. Slowly but surely all my symptoms went away and today I can eat like a normal person! No more elemental formula and no more sickness. No more antibiotics, just real food as medicine.

I recommend friends and family to Dr. Cabral who have all had the same success with their own health issues. He knows what he's doing and what he does works. I'm now weaning off the supplements and my body has been able to heal itself! I travel, do yoga, work, and have a life again thanks to Dr. Cabral."

- Alexis P.

FROM ADRENAL FATIGUE TO FANTASTIC!

Dr. Cabral is without a doubt the most knowledgeable, understanding and kind doctor I have ever met. I feel I found him just in time, as I was at my breaking point with feeling so sick and anxious all of the time. It's 5 months later now, and I am like a different person. I am thinner, calmer, more energetic and obviously healthier and happier than I ever could have imagined! I don't believe another doctor would have been able to help as Dr Cabral has! He's the best!

- Judith K.

SHRUNK MY TROUBLE AREAS

"I really wanted to lose weight from my trouble areas that no matter how much I work out or try to eat healthy I never seem to be able to. By the end (of my detox) I loved how I felt. I had more energy and I LOVED how my body transformed. I now have a thigh gap which seems like a silly thing to say, but I haven't had one in years and I could actually feel how my thighs had gotten smaller when I walk…"

- Alyssa B

Table of Contents

Introduction ································ xix
My Mission ·································· xxiii
How to Use this Book ·························· xxvii

Part 1: The Current State of Our World ············ 1
Discover the Top 10 Toxins and how they are keeping you from getting well, losing weight, and feeling alive again!
What Happened to Our World? ····················· 3
Toxic Enemy #1 Heavy Metals ····················· 11
Toxic Enemy #2 Synthetic Food ···················· 24
Toxic Enemy #3 Pesticides & DDT ·················· 32
Toxic Enemy #4 Tap Water ······················· 38
Toxic Enemy #5 Stress ··························· 44
Toxic Enemy #6 Electrosmog ······················ 49
Toxic Enemy #7 Home Sick ······················· 54
Toxic Enemy #8 Skin Care Products ················ 59
Toxic Enemy #9 Pharmaceuticals ··················· 68
Toxic Enemy #10 Gut Bugs ······················· 74

Part 2: The Rain Barrel Effect ···················· 81
The *Rain Barrel Effect* is revealed. Find out how it holds the missing key to finally getting well again. This chapter will also explain how you got to where you are right now.
The Real Reason We Become Sick, Tired, & Overweight ·········· 83

The RBE Toxicity Quiz · 117
How Full Is Your Rain Barrel? · 119
Now that you know what the Top 10 Toxic Enemies are that surround us and what the *Rain Barrel Effect* is, it's time to take the toxicity quiz and find out *"how full is your rain barrel?"*

Part 3: The Search for Answers · · · · · · · · · · · · · · · · · · · 129
Although by now I had finished my Doctorate in Naturopathy I still hadn't found the "missing link" to reversing dis-ease, weight gain, and rapid aging. My search describes how I discovered the answers I was searching for and now share with the world…
A Skeptic's Journey · 131

Part 4: The DESTRESS Protocol · · · · · · · · · · · · · · · · · · 153
After discovering the time-tested secrets to getting well I had to create a formula that could be used by anyone, anywhere in the world. My DESTRESS Protocol™ in this section walks you through the exact process I use in my private practice:
Diet · 155
Exercise · 179
Stress Reduction · 190
Toxins: Part 1 How to Remove, Reduce, and Eliminate Environmental Toxins in Your Life · · · · · · · · · · · · · · 216
Toxins: Part 2 How to Remove, Reduce, and Eliminate Environmental Toxins in Your Body · · · · · · · · · · · · · 239
Rest · 260
Toxic Emotions · 281
Supplements · 310
Success (Mindset) · 333
The Dr. Cabral Detox Manual · · · · · · · · · · · · · · · · · · · 355
The Best Time To Start · 384

PART 5: 21 Days to Your New Life ·XXX
I believe in helping people get a quick win and start seeing results right away. This quick start section contains the manual I use to help people get well, lose weight, and feel alive again within just 21 days.

Part 6: Appendix & Resources · XXX
It's Time to Begin

    About the Author · 391
    RBE Success Resources & Recommendations · · · · · · · · · · · · · · · · 393
    Resources · 397

Introduction

When Sara came to me she had run out of places to turn...

She had no other options.

And at this point she had nothing to lose but she was still skeptical.

It's not exactly how I prefer to start off an initial consultation, but I certainly understood her frustration. After all, I was once in her same position.

She had been lied to, given an inaccurate picture of her health, and as a result, she was suffering. She couldn't eat anything without becoming extremely bloated and she fluctuated between bouts of severe constipation and diarrhea.

But lately, Sara's more pressing complaints revolved around brain fog, fatigue, anxiety, low drive, and decreased ambition. She said that her workouts were flat and not enjoyable and that this pretty much described the rest of her life as well.

She also had a great boyfriend whom she lived with, but she complained that her libido was so low she didn't even want to be touched. Plus, she felt like she was constantly swollen, retaining water, and had gained another 10 pounds even though she was mostly "eating healthily" and doing 60-minutes of exercise most days a week.

As she vented and I listened intently for another 20-minutes, I could sense that this was probably the first-time Sara had actually had the opportunity to lay everything out on the table about what had been going on with her over the past few years.

You could see a look of relief in her face to be vocalizing this finally, but at the same time her years of struggle and disappointment were obvious.

She had seen dozens of other doctors, GI specialists, and alternative health practitioners who could give her no lasting relief, except maybe a week or two reprieve from the misery she endured, before she would find herself right back in the same state of poor health.

She was extremely frustrated at having spent tens of thousands of dollars on treatments, supplements, and appointments only to be let down time and time again. After such a big investment, who could blame her.

Unfortunately, Sara's story isn't unique. This is the state of our current healthcare system and because of it, people like Sara suffer needlessly every day as a result.

But there is hope…

No one needs to be a victim of a broken system, constantly shuffled from doctor to doctor, put on one cocktail after another of medications that bring no relief, only to be told there is nothing left they can do to help in the end.

Like Sara, I too have a similar story. It's not pleasant and it brings up painful memories every time I recall it, but because of that low point in my life, I have made it my mission to ensure that others do not have to suffer *if they choose not to.*

In the coming chapters I will share my full story with you and I'll also reveal Sara's new life.

But for now, I want you to know that I wrote the *Rain Barrel Effect* to explain how we all get sick, overweight, and begin to break down. I also wrote this book so that you will know *you can* get well and *you will* once you understand one very specific factor:

Your body has an innate power to heal itself once you allow it to return to a state of equilibrium. It is only an imbalance in one of the systems of your body that causes you to struggle with the symptoms of "dis-ease." (I will refer to disease as "dis-ease" throughout this book since diseases are nothing more than a name we give to a collection of symptoms that we then are told to mask with drugs.)

Getting well, losing weight, and turning back the clock on aging is not a mystery, yet the truth has been hidden for so many years. It took me over a decade of study and travel all over the world to find those answers. Now I'd like to share with you what I discovered, so that together we can help you live the life you've always wanted.

Let the healing begin -

Dr. Stephen Cabral
Doctor of Naturopathy
Ayurvedic & Functional Medicine Practitioner

My Mission

Before I share with you the condensed version of 20 years of research in natural health and medicine, as well as the information and lessons gathered over 250,000 successful client appointments who finally discovered health, weight loss, and restored energy, I would like to start at the beginning…

As a kid growing up, I never saw myself becoming a doctor.

I wanted to be an archeologist who traveled all over the world exploring ancient mysteries, studying lost civilizations, and unearthing long buried secrets.

I studied hard in school, got good grades, and exceled at sports until one day all of that was taken away from me. I woke up one Monday morning, so deathly ill that my life changed forever.

Had I known what I know now, I could have stopped myself from getting so very sick. And after having learned how to heal myself, I could no longer sit back and watch the same symptoms begin placing others in a state of poor health, when I knew what was causing it and how to fix it.

In the next chapter, you will get your first glimpse into why we are all becoming so sick, run down, depressed, exhausted, and imbalanced. You will also learn about the *Rain Barrel Effect* and how this concept relates directly to how dis-ease develops in the body, as well as how we can reverse and heal from these dis-eases.

Right now, the air you breathe, the water you drink, the food you eat, the clothes you wear, and the chair you sit in are exposing you to more toxic chemicals than your body knows what to do with.

It's a slow poisoning of your body's systems. These systems were never genetically designed for this type of toxic onslaught.

Did you know that there are over 77,000 man-made chemicals in the environment all around you?[1] Did you also know it is these very same chemicals that have been proven to cause cancer, disease, and weight gain?

With these types of data-driven facts, it becomes easy to see why cancer is becoming the #1 cause of death in the world and will soon affect every 1 out of 2 people.[2]

But it doesn't stop there.

These chemicals in our environment are a tremendous source of inflammation in our body. And this inflammation then leads to a host of issues such as auto-immune responses, skin problems, blood pressure issues, cardiovascular disease, fatigue, digestive distress, brain fog, and many more.

Just look at a few of the latest US health statistics:

- Auto-immune disease affects 50 million people[3]
- Every 1 in 4 deaths in the U.S. is due to cardiovascular disease[4]
- High blood pressure affects 1 in 3 people[5]
- 13% of the U.S. population suffer with debilitating migraines[6]
- Anxiety or mood disorders afflict over 40 million people[7]
- Obesity affects 1 in 3 people and 2 out of 3 people are overweight[8]

There is no coincidence here. We spend more each and every year on healthcare, yet people are getting more and more sick. And to make matters worse, it's now estimated that the next generation of children will be the first to die younger than their parents.[9]

Our medical system has no answers except develop and patent more pharmaceutical drugs. But are drugs really the answer? Unless you believe treating the outward symptoms of a disease is actually doing anything other than covering up a ticking time-bomb, I'd have to say no.

Therefore, I see no other choice but for all of us to take our health care back into our own hands.

It doesn't have to be scary or difficult. I firmly believe that once you are shown how easy it can be to remove all the toxins your body is storing, rebalance your system, and replenish your vital reserves, you may actually begin to enjoy the process.

I believe most people want to be well. They don't want to suffer. They want more energy, vitality, and, most of all, they want to feel alive!

They simply haven't been given the full picture of how to pull it all together.

This is why when I first met Sara she had no idea what she could possibly do next. She thought she had tried it all. What was holding her back was the same belief that most of us cling to – the idea that we must always be adding more to our body or our life, not taking things away.

Once I helped her focus on elimination and removal, her health was soon restored.

I have the privilege of seeing people in my practice get well every day and recover long after they and their doctors had previously given up hope. I want the same for you. I want you to begin enjoying life again without ever having to worry about how your health or weight is holding you back from what you want in life.

You deserve that.

Now let's show you how to get it.

How to Use this Book

Shock and disbelief.

That's usually the reaction I get when I first explain the reason why most of us are in poor health and experience suffering.

The reason for this is that big corporations from the media, to the pharmaceutical industry, to the government, to food manufacturers – all these huge earning entities that are strictly profit-driven earn endless amounts of money as long as things stay the way they are. They do not want you to know what I'm about to share with you.

Because if too many people find out this information, then perhaps a shift in the public mindset will occur and with it, their profits may see a down shift too.

So they have a very vested interest in keeping you in the dark. But make no mistake about it – a movement has already begun.

Many health-conscious individuals and families all over the world have started saying *no* to drugs and *yes* to a life of health and prosperity in every sense of the word.

It is my goal that, for the first time ever, you will discover the true root cause for the sickness and dis-ease you may needlessly suffer from.

I also want the information that you're about to receive to be written in a conversational manner, so that you can best absorb it and then put it into action. This book is written for anyone to be able to read, apply, and get results.

With that goal in mind, I broke the *Rain Barrel Effect* up into sections:

PART 1

The first part of this book will most likely bring out a mixed bag of emotions where you begin to question much of what you've been led to believe about the world constructed around you. You may even question how or why these things could possibly happen. I asked myself those very same questions when I first discovered the hidden truth.

However, it's important to know what we're up against on our quest to be well, take back our bodies, and live longer and stronger lives. This is why I share this information. I want you to be fully awake with your eyes wide open in a world where being healthy & happy is no longer the norm. What I don't want you to be is overwhelmed – There is an answer and by the time you finish the book you will have it.

PART 2

Once we lay out what to watch out for in Part 1, I will then very clearly break down exactly how we get sick, fat, and unhappy. I'll show you that no disease sets in overnight. Since this may be the first time you're hearing this I'm also going to explain it in real world talk, just as if you and I were having a conversation together. It is in this chapter that you will discover what the *Rain Barrel Effect* is all about.

PART 3

In this section I recount my travels overseas and how it wasn't until I left the US, that I finally discovered the "secret" of how to get truly well again.

This is more than just normalizing your lab test levels. It is a deep sense of well-being that only comes from bringing your body back to a rejuvenated state. This state is a complete balance between body and mind and it is the answer we've all been searching for.

PART 4

In Part 4, I'll share with you the exact plan I use every day in my Functional Medicine practice to help people just like you finally get well, lose weight, and feel alive again! It blends the best of modern-day medicine and the ancient healing forms. It's called the DESTRESS Protocol™ and it's something you can begin to implement immediately right at home to start seeing the benefits in your life!

One additional item I added to each DESTRESS Protocol™ chapter is a "cheat sheet" or action plan at the end. It represents what I believe to be the easiest way to getting started.

PART 5

For the first time ever, I'm going to give away the exact 21-day Dr. Cabral Detox manual I've been using for over 5 years with people all over the world to help them rebalance their body (and mind).

It is simply the fastest and easiest way to jumpstart your results. If you do nothing else, this protocol will walk you step-by-step through the healing process.

PART 6

At the end of this book, I will provide you with an easy to use resource appendix full of helpful tips, products, websites, bonuses, and recipe guides. It will dramatically shorten your time needed to return your body back to the state of health it was meant to live in.

Plus, these resources will save you money and the time needed to do all the research yourself. Also, you will see this mentioned throughout the book, but for every resource listed in this book simply go to: *StephenCabral.com/rbe*

That one resource page contains *everything* you need.

REAL WORLD RESULTS FOR REAL PEOPLE

You should also know that the *Rain Barrel Effect* was at one time a 700+ page book heavily focused on the science of how your body becomes sick, overweight, and diseased.

However, after realizing that this format might not be the best way to help people the most, I reduced the technical aspects of the science and research data studies to be footnotes and asterisks – This allows those who are interested to do additional reading on their own.

I believe this final format is a lot more fun, approachable, and action-oriented to help you get the results you're looking for!

It's going to be an amazing journey and my hope and belief for you is that by the end of this book, you'll feel a sense of relief. I want you to know you have arrived – that this book holds the answer and the plan you've been searching for in order to get your mind, body, and health back.

It is now with immense gratitude that I bring you the *Rain Barrel Effect*.

Part 1
The Current State of Our World

What Happened to Our World?

"1 in 2 will get cancer in their lifetime…"

- BRITISH JOURNAL OF CANCER, 2015

Every second of every day, more and more people are being diagnosed with debilitating diseases of all kinds.

And no one is safe. Women, children, and men of all ages have more than doubled their risk for deadly diseases, most of them incurable, and are firmly shackled to a lifetime of poor health.

The grim truth is that your risk factor for getting cancer, diabetes or heart disease is now close to 1 in 2.

That means in the United States alone, literally half of all adults will get cancer unless something changes. The problem is nothing is changing.

To make matters worse, chronic health conditions and autoimmune disorders of all types are on the rise and affect approximately 50 million people, just in the United States.[1]

Alzheimer's has more than doubled since 1980, and other mental health disorders affect millions without any clear sign of how to combat them.[2]

CURRENT ODDS OF DEVELOPING DISEASE

- 1 in 2 men will get cancer, 1 in 3 women will as well[3]
- 1 in 3 will develop diabetes by 2050. Currently, 1 in 10 already have diabetes.[4]
- 1 in 3 will develop heart disease[5]
- 1 in 4 will be diagnosed with arthritis[6]
- 1 in 5 will develop some form of autoimmune disease

This is a worldwide problem. However, the United States, even as the top spender in healthcare costs, is ranked near the bottom of all developed nations for quality of human health.

The U.S. spends more but with little results

THE FAILED HEALTHCARE SYSTEM

Health Care Spending as a Percentage of GDP, 1980–2013

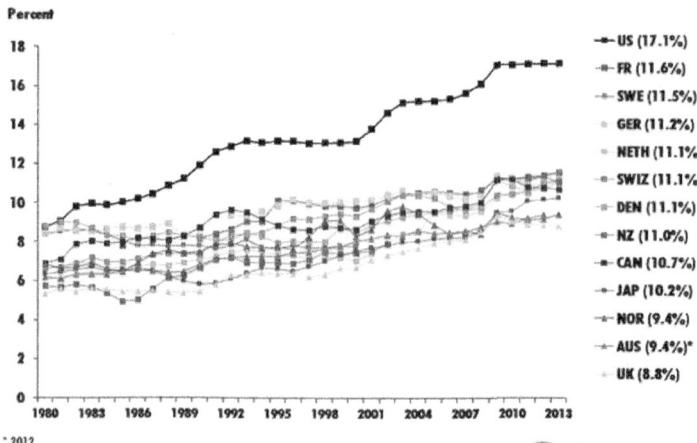

- US (17.1%)
- FR (11.6%)
- SWE (11.5%)
- GER (11.2%)
- NETH (11.1%)
- SWIZ (11.1%)
- DEN (11.1%)
- NZ (11.0%)
- CAN (10.7%)
- JAP (10.2%)
- NOR (9.4%)
- AUS (9.4%)*
- UK (8.8%)

* 2012.
Notes: GDP refers to gross domestic product. Dutch and Swiss data are for current spending only, and exclude spending on capital formation of health care providers.
Source: OECD Health Data 2015.

The COMMONWEALTH FUND

(The chart above depicts each nation's healthcare spending and the graph below ranks each country by their health.)

Notice that although the U.S. spends more than any other country per person on healthcare, it is still ranked 37th in terms of overall quality of health by the World Health Organization (WHO).[7]

BEST TO WORST HEALTH RANKINGS

1. France
2. Italy
3. San Marino
4. Andorra
5. Malta
6. Singapore
7. Spain
8. Oman
9. Austria
10. Japan
11. Norway
12. Portugal
13. Monaco
14. Greece
15. Iceland
16. Luxembourg
17. Netherlands
18. United Kingdom
19. Ireland
20. Switzerland
21. Belgium
22. Colombia
23. Sweden
24. Cyprus
25. Germany
26. Saudi Arabia
27. United Arab Emirates
28. Israel
29. Morocco
30. Canada
31. Finland
32. Australia
33. Chile
34. Denmark
35. Dominica
36. Costa Rica
37. U.S.A

DISEASES OF OLD AGE

As bad as the statistics are for individuals living in industrialized nations with good healthcare systems in place, what's even more frightening is that these numbers include children.

You see, the argument for spending more on healthcare and the escalating rates of people dying from cancer and other diseases at record numbers is often explained away by doctors as being due to the fact that people live longer today than they ever have, but this simply is not true.

Our children are now being diagnosed with Rheumatoid arthritis, obesity, type 2 diabetes, and many other health conditions that were at one time reserved only for the adult population.

And as I stated in our opening chapter, children born after 2014 will be the first generation predicted to die at a younger age than their parents will.[8]

These life-threatening childhood health conditions don't even include the fact that ADHD, autism, dyslexia, and other learning disabilities have increased in children dramatically over the past few decades.

Did you know that 1 out of every 68 children born is now on the Autism spectrum? That's an unprecedented 30% rise in just 2 years. This is up from just 1 in 2,000 children in the 1980's being diagnosed as being on the Autism spectrum[9]

Even if you argue quantitatively that there has been an increase in diagnoses alone, as more teachers, school officials, and parents are becoming educated about signs and symptoms of autism, you simply can't deny the dramatic increase in cases of the disorder with that thin explanation alone.

As a parent of two young girls, I was also disturbed to read the research on how the average fetus is exposed to as many as 287 harmful chemicals that can cause anything from birth defects, to learning disabilities, to cancer.[10]

The umbilical cord itself, which supplies blood and nutrients to the unborn child can often contain close to double the amount of heavy metals like mercury than the mother contains in her own blood. In fact, the umbilical cords of newborns typically contain over 100 toxins, cancerous chemicals, and heavy metals, such as mercury, cadmium, or lead.[11]

As a father and naturopath, this worries me. How many toxins are my children exposed to at school or at their carefully manicured playgrounds?

This is our new reality.

The bottom-line is that health issues of all kinds are on the rise at historic rates and no one offers a good explanation.

It's not that any one researcher, scientist, or doctor doesn't want to figure out what is at work in the world suddenly causing this rapid rise in disease, it's that there is not one clear-cut answer.

Rather, it is a compounding of many different factors that has led us down this path. This is why one silver bullet approach will never provide the answer we're looking for.

THE ANSWER LIES IN HOW WE GOT HERE

When scientists want to create cancer (or a brain disease) in a lab rat for experimental research they expose that rat to a common food pesticide. This pesticide, in turn, causes cancer in the rodent that researchers can then try various experiments to try to cure that cancer.

When I first read this bit of scientific data I was shocked.

I understand the value of research and trying to cure the world's most insidious diseases, but shouldn't we hit the rewind button and study the pesticide that gave the rat cancer in the first place?

Although it's not common knowledge, the world's leading health organizations have stated that 95% of all cancer is diet and environment related.[12]

This literally means at least 95 out of 100 cancer cases could have been prevented. Stated another way, 95 out of every 100 cancer cases is man-made and is caused by living in a cancerous environment.

As you'll see in a moment, we're not just talking about cancer.

The vast majority of all health conditions are lifestyle related.

Even autoimmune diseases, which I'll be discussing momentarily, have less to do with genetics and far more to do with gut dysbiosis, which has been connected to over 90% of all cases of autoimmune disorders.[13]

Of course, this gut dysbiosis (imbalanced intestinal bacteria) comes from all the toxins we inhale and the toxins we ingest from pesticide tainted crops as well.

So, although I'm not against promoting scientific research for the benefit of curing diseases when someone is suffering, what I am suggesting is that our scientific radar might be pointed in the wrong direction entirely.

NAVIGATING AN UNCLEAN WORLD

Now that we know how much all diseases, mental and physical, are on the rise, it's time to talk about *why*.

Many of the commonly diagnosed diseases today, especially diabetes and cancer, are mainly a product of modern society. This means our current condition was essentially manufactured over the past 60-70 years.

In the grand scheme of things, mankind has been around for millennia, whether you are an evolutionist or creationist. Yet we've had this huge explosion in diseases that were quite rare in just the past few decades.

Why? Well, let's ask what changed about society...

In this case, we can see a direct correlation with the industrialization of countries and a decline in health and we can definitely argue without a doubt that some drastic environmental changes must have occurred.

And we know it must have to do with industrialization, pollutions, and a general toxification of the environment because these diseases are most widespread in developed countries and across all populations rather than in specific populations.

This leads us to the conclusion that there is a widespread systemic environmental issue that is affecting everyone. I am not the first person to see this correlation.

There are many studies for you to choose from to chart this direct correlation between environmental toxins and a subsequent worsening of human health and I will be highlighting a few in a moment.

These harsh chemical toxins are ones we are all exposed to most every day of our lives and because of this, our chances for developing a deadly array of diseases and cancers increases drastically with every year that passes.

The good news is that we can reduce our exposure to toxins by becoming more aware of the worst ones and minimizing or avoiding exposure to them altogether.

Better yet, we can work to remove most of these cancer and disease-causing chemicals from our body!

AWARENESS IS THE ANSWER

This is why it's crucial we understand:

    a. How toxic the world truly is
    b. How toxins get into our bodies
    c. Where the worst ones come from
    d. How to reduce toxic exposure and eradicate toxins from our lives and homes, as much as possible
    e. Learn about heavy metal and chemical detoxification methods and how to restore health to the system

It's only when you understand the threat and strategize a way to defeat it that true victory can be yours.

Now let's review the most pervasive and damaging toxins in the environment and how they affect our health.

THE TOP 10 TOXINS

What we've accepted as normal is anything but that.

As you're about to see, some of the most dangerous toxins in the world have made their way into almost all commercial water, food, household cleaners, and products of all kinds including air conditioner filters, carpeting, hair spray, de-icers on subways, pesticides at the park, chlorine in your swimming pool, dechlorinating products in your water, as well as fluoride and other dangerous chemicals. This doesn't even include personal care products of all kinds. Plus, they're also in the air we breathe – especially if you live near a city and most definitely if you live near a factory.

Note: As you're reading over these common, but well disguised toxins that you may come into contact with every day, I do not want you to lose hope or become overwhelmed. Remember, we can only protect ourselves and our loved ones when we know the enemy and have the proper information to resist!

Now let's review the Top 10 Toxic Enemies to watch out for:

Toxic Enemy #1
Heavy Metals

> *"For each 1,000 lbs. of environmentally released mercury, there was a 61% increase in ASD (Autism). The same study showed an increase of 43% in the rate of special education rates..."*
>
> - UNIVERSITY OF TEXAS[14]

Heavy metal toxicity is one of the most overlooked causes for disease, neurological diseases and disorders, and reproductive problems.

I want to devote some special attention, here, to heavy metal toxicity because no one is talking about this with the anger or passion they should be. Every person that gets tested today tests for an array of toxic loads from various heavy metals that fall just shy of poisonous.

Heavy metals wreak havoc on our body at a cellular level and they cause massive inflammation as well, triggering autoimmune reactions and diseases while placing us at risk for a complete domino effect of diseases to follow.

Heavy metals quite literally corrode your body from the inside out. Let's begin with why you should be concerned about your level of heavy metal accumulation.

When exposed to an *acute* dose of heavy metals – a one time dose, that is - the immediate symptoms you could experience are:

- nausea
- cramping
- dizziness
- sweating
- headaches
- difficulty breathing
- impaired thinking and motor control

However, the real problem with heavy metal toxicity isn't typically with one acute high-dose exposure. It's from a lifetime of leaching exposure through our waters, soil, the foods we eat, the vaccinations we receive, medicines we ingest, and air that we breathe.

Over time, as heavy metals build up in your system—their effects actually mimic the symptoms of other diseases that we attribute them to like chronic fatigue, fibromyalgia, autism, depression – could it be these diseases never would have manifested in human populations without heavy metals being introduced into our food, water, and air?

Gradual heavy metal toxicity will mimic many of the diseases we give names to; diseases we quickly diagnose and prescribe something for to mask the symptoms.

Here are some common symptoms of lower-level *chronic* heavy metal toxicity:

- fatigue
- joint pain
- muscle weakness
- poor mood & depression

- learning disabilities
- hyperactivity & anxiety
- dysregulated blood sugar
- digestive issues & low absorption
- reproductive problems & birth defects

When you look at those longer-term exposure symptoms, you can clearly see that many people suffering from mystery illnesses like chronic fatigue, fibromyalgia, Lyme disease symptoms, IBS, Crohn's, ADHD, and major depressive disorder, may actually have a heavy metal toxic burden or other toxicity as one of the real root causes of their symptoms.

What kind of heavy metal toxicity is most common today? Well, let's talk about the most common heavy metals in our environment. Some of these you can avoid and some are not so easy to avoid. They are in our air and may even be leaching through the concrete poured for our basements, coming through the soil and gradually penetrating cement to toxify our homes.

MERCURY

Mercury is often implicated as one of the most dangerous heavy metals to mankind since it can damage both your brain and body fairly quickly if you're exposed to too much of it.

Mercury is found in thousands of common items like contact lens solutions, nasal sprays, prescription drugs, vaccines, flu shots, fungicides, pesticides, fertilizers, as well as from industrial smokestacks spewing it into the air we breathe.

This means the run off from these factories infect nearly everything we consume that grows from our soil, air, and seas. This is also why it's so crucial to be weary of what type of fish you are consuming, as well as the quantity.

The larger predatory fish to watch out for when trying to avoid mercury are tuna, swordfish, shark, tilefish, and bluefish.

These types of fish are going to be very high on the mercury list and by eating them often you will then begin to accumulate more and more mercury in your system. *(A full list of high/low mercury fish will be provided in the resource section.)*

I remember the first time I ran a Hair Tissue Mineral Analysis test when I was in college, trying to cure myself of a debilitating dis-ease, and was amazed and frightened when my mercury levels scored off the charts.

My functional medicine doctor asked me if I was eating a lot of fish, to which I replied, "I eat canned tuna almost every day." Back then, I was into natural bodybuilding and I thought that was the best way to get in a lot of high quality safe protein. It turns out that is definitely not the case…

Another common exposure to mercury is through having oder cavity fillings, known as "silver" dental amalgams. Those metal fillings contain toxic levels of mercury, which can damage every facet of your health.

This means that every time you chew food, micro doses of mercury may be released into your bloodstream. In fact, what's leaching into your gums can go right to your heart.

The tricky thing is that if you *do* decide to have them removed, it must be done safely by a holistically trained biological dentist. This takes additional schooling since it is not taught as part of the standard dental education.

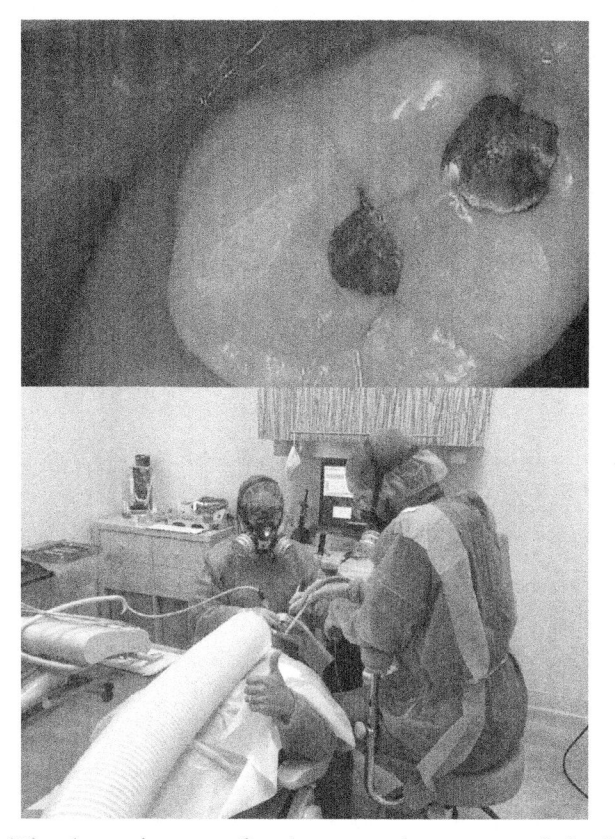

(The photos above are of me having my last 2 mercury"silver" amalgams removed by Dr. Yuko Torigoe in Boston, MA.)

You can find safe mercury amalgam-removal trained dentists at https://iaomt.org.

One last note on mercury is that if you're thinking about getting pregnant or you have a child with a learning disorder, or you have some type of health issue yourself, you may want to consider getting tested and at least cutting back on your exposure. I will provide a list of qualified Functional Medicine doctors in your area and at-home lab testing options in the resource section of this book.

ALUMINUM

Aluminum is one of the most pervasive heavy metals today on Earth. It's also one that can easily cause toxic overload, which often results in nervous system damage (MS & ALS), DNA genetic replication disruptions, and neurological health issues (Parkinson's, Alzheimer's, dementia, memory loss).

The reason aluminum has become such an issue these past few decades is that it's found in anti-perspirants, cosmetics, antacids, cans, vaccines, dental work, cookware, and even tap water. If you're like most people today, you're likely being exposed to aluminum multiple times per day.

In one of the coming chapters on toxins (Part 4), I will present you with some easy to use charts and graphs of how to replace the common high aluminum products you're currently using with much healthier alternatives.

As a Functional Medicine practitioner, one of my main concerns with aluminum is its implication in neurological issues. The average person is now taking in between 30-50mg of aluminum a day and much of that is through aluminum silicates that are in the air and attached to dust particles, which then get absorbed directly into the olfactory nerve and right into the olfactory bulb in the brain.[15]

Truthfully, the aluminum vapors in the tap water coming out of your shower and faucet are one of the most concerning ways in which you are exposed to this metal. In fact, the heavy metal tainted vapors we inhale as we're showering are much more toxic than those in the water hitting our skin.

Vapor allows these toxins to immediately enter the bloodstream, where it flows to all the organs and tissues, doing excessive damage everywhere it goes, including the brain.

Heavy metals like to deposit themselves in tissues, especially fat tissue. And our brain if full of fatty tissue. This is why all heavy metals are toxic. They build up and store in our body and poison us from within. In fact, inhaling aluminum via vapor has been shown to increase your risk for Alzheimer's by as much as 300%.

Although I no longer believe it's possible to avoid aluminum completely, it's vitally important to lower your daily aluminum exposure in order to reduce your risk of all types of disease and neurological degeneration.

We will review how to do that in coming chapters and I'll be providing you with some easy-to-install shower and bath filters to capture the aluminum (and chlorine) before you or your children breathe it in.

CADMIUM

The reason I decided to include cadmium is that it can cause:

- Cancer
- Kidney disease
- Neurological issues
- High blood pressure
- Arteriosclerosis
- Reproductive defects[16]

Cadmium is one of the lesser known heavy metals and is found predominantly in our soil. It gets transferred into many grains, potatoes, tobacco and other vegetables. It's also found in higher levels in organ meats like kidney and liver.

Aside from foods, cadmium is found in some fertilizers, batteries, ceramics, nail polish, rubber tires, plastics, paints and pesticides. Cadmium can also be found in drinking water and air.

Like many other heavy metals, it can displace other beneficial minerals within our body. In the case of cadmium, it can replace calcium in your bones, leading to greater chances of osteoporosis or other bone disorders.

Cadmium can also stimulate your adrenal cortex, leading to greater stress levels and high cortisol. This, in turn, can displace magnesium and increase sodium retention leading to symptoms of high blood pressure and anxiety.

This is one more reason why treating adrenal issues isn't as easy as giving them a "boost."

An additional side effect of high cadmium levels is that it can block zinc absorption in the intestines and, thus, cause conditions that affects the muscles, gut, immunity, or tissue repair. This includes a hardening of the arteries and other cardiovascular-based issues due to increased calcium deposits.

I hope at this point you're beginning to see how everything we call a "disease" has its root problem in much deeper imbalances and toxicities within the body.

LEAD

While heavy metal toxicity from lead is far less prevalent today than it was decades ago, it can still cause a host of issues when someone is exposed to lead, especially in high doses or at a young age.

Homes or buildings constructed before 1978 in the United States can still contain lead based paint that can deteriorate and cause unknown lead exposure. Children and pregnant women exposed to paint chips or lead dust particles in the air are at increased risk for complications from lead including birth defects, seizures, and even learning disabilities.

Lead can also be found in pipes, specialty paint, toys, ammunition, ground water, batteries, pottery, crafts, construction material, and some cosmetics.

While the amount of lead used in home and building construction has decreased over time, it is still devastating to the nervous system and cardiovascular functionality.

I recently worked with a man named Jim who had multiple unexplained symptoms resulting in an inability to walk due to excruciating pain and major swelling in his legs.

He went to specialist after specialist, all of whom kept searching for cancer. They finally gave up and told him they really had no answers to his problems.

By the time I met Jim he was pale, on crutches, and unable to stand for more than a few minutes at a time. He often fell asleep right in his chair as we were talking due to extreme exhaustion.

After spending some time reviewing all of Jim's blood work and labs, I could see how from a functional medicine perspective that there was a lot wrong.

I didn't believe he had cancer for multiple reasons. He had very healthy white blood cell counts, for example. Many other biomarkers for health were extremely high too.

But clearly, this man's body was shutting down fast and we needed to do something to help him…

My initial suspicion, after seeing hundreds of Jim's lab data points, was that he had all the indicators, such as a lowered red blood cell count, of blood clots or internal bleeding somewhere. However these indicators could also be a symptom of a possible lead toxicity or infection.

I ran more tests and found all of the above initial health concerns to be true. After more combing through Jim's files and questioning, I discovered that Jim had worked for the city water department for decades, and had been exposed to lead pipes and ground water on a near daily basis. He also had been injured just weeks before that when a piece of equipment had fallen on his leg.

With a plan in place we were able to detox his body from the lead, fortify his missing minerals and vitamins and rebuild his blood to healthy levels. Jim is now back on his feet, is down 36 lbs., his blood work looks fantastic, and he's finally feeling well again!

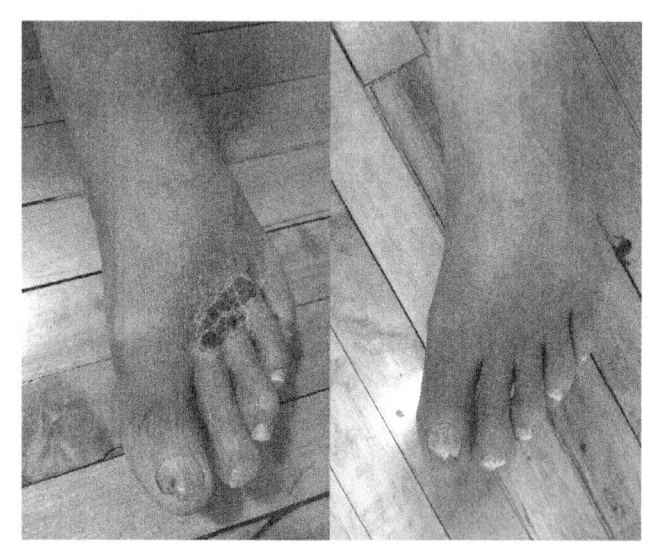

(Jim's before and after photos are an incredible example of how the human body can heal when it is given what it needs to remove toxins and rebalance itself.)

ARSENIC

Like all heavy metals that accumulate in the body, arsenic can derange genetic material, cause cancer, and hundreds of health issues affecting the blood vessels, nervous system, brain, gut, skin, lungs, and reproductive organs.

Although arsenic is naturally occurring and is a part of the earth's crust (like other heavy metals), its intake should be avoided.

Arsenic exposure can come from both organic and inorganic compounds, but we are mainly exposed to arsenic from our food and water sources.

Smokers will inhale more arsenic due to the fact that it is one of the hundreds of chemicals contained in cigarette smoke.

Arsenic also turns up in some other odd places such as chemotherapy treatments for acute promyelocytic leukemia and other cancers.[17]

It was formerly used in some herbicides, fungicides, and pesticides, which still remain in our earth's soil and contaminate our current food supply.

Additionally, arsenic can make its way into the ocean from coal-burning power plants and their toxic smoke. It then pollutes waters and allows crustaceans and other bottom feeders like lobsters, crabs, clams, oysters, scallops, and mussels to absorb higher levels of arsenic as well.

Unfortunately, any man-made creation can contain high levels of heavy metals. Just look at your own children's parks and playgrounds. The preservative they use on the wooden structures contains copper chromated arsenate, which helps to seal and keep the wood from deteriorating. It can also make us sick with repeated exposure…

Again, this is not to scare you, but rather to impress upon you the true cause for why we are seeing a massive spike in almost all health-related issues.

I also want to reiterate that all arsenic exposure will not be totally avoidable due to it naturally occurring in ground water which then feeds our plants, and in turn, the animals who eat the plants. One of the most common food items typically containing high levels of arsenic is rice.

There are many theories as to why, which include the former use of lead arsenate in fertilizer for cotton fields, former chicken feed contains arsenic, and general contamination of crops through high arsenic watering. However, being aware of this potential contamination is the first step in avoiding overconsumption of arsenic. You can find low-arsenic rice through brands such as Lundberg and Lotus.

Being well informed and making choices based in awareness is what will allow us to continue living in this modern world while still protecting our health and wellbeing. I feel comfortable eating rice from the less toxic varieties, just like I do occasionally eating fish with low levels of mercury.

We're living in a highly toxic and polluted environment, but the solution isn't just to pretend it's not there. But, we also must be realistic.

And, of course, I will provide you with exactly what I use for my myself, my family, and those I care for in my Functional Medicine practice in Part 4 under the DESTRESS Protocol™.

BROMINES

While there are numerous heavy metals that could be discussed in this book, I obviously can't review every one in just a chapter's worth of data.

However, I did feel it was important to share the harmful effects of bromines with you. Specifically, because this element is hardly ever talked about, but it lies at the bottom of numerous unexplained health conditions.

Bromines are typically found in pools, water, medicines, and common processed food items. Bromines are used every day as an additive to breads to help the yeast rise, even though it is well known to be highly toxic to humans!

And like most other synthetic products, it too is one of the heavy metals found in everyday items like curtains, chair coverings, sofas, and computer screens.

And thus it is difficult, if not impossible, to avoid.

Although not well known, bromine accumulation is also one of the hidden causes of skin, eye, and throat issues at both an acute and chronic level.

I've worked with several people with unexplained red dots on the skin called "cherry angiomas," and other so called "age-related" marks that have been directly attributed to elevated bromine levels.

Also, if you're suffering from low thyroid or Hashimoto's disease, bromine could be responsible. The reason for this is that your thyroid needs iodine as one of its essential nutrients and bromines displace iodine and therefore, your thyroid function lowers.

This in turn slows your metabolism, causes weight gain, and a host of other unwanted low mood, low energy, low vitality disorders.

The good news is that like the other heavy metals I've discussed today, bromines can be eliminated from your body quickly and painlessly.

This detoxification allows your body to begin to heal without having to constantly deal with the internal threats from heavy metals that disrupt your nervous, immune, and endocrine system.

Now it's time to move onto our next toxic enemy, which is added directly to our food supply. Unfortunately, most consumers have no idea what's going on every time they take a bite of what looks like a "normal" meal…

Toxic Enemy #2
Synthetic Food

> *"Milk and dairy now contain up to 10X the amount of IGF-1 growth hormone linked to prostate, colon, and other types of cancer."*
>
> - AMERICAN CANCER SOCIETY

Now that we've revealed the hidden dangers associated with heavy metal overload, I want to switch gears and talk more about how genetically modified organisms (GMOs) and other changes to our natural foods are causing a predicable decline in our health.

One of the reasons why food is such an important part of our health is because as humans, we literally consume between 30-50 tons of food in our lifetime.

It can be the largest factor in whether we maintain robust optimal wellness or a life ridden with dis-ease and despair. The reason for this is that food is meant to give us life, energy, and vitality. However, what we've done to our food supply directly contradicts its intended purpose.

I will be talking more about which foods to avoid and which ones to eat in abundance in the coming section on "Diet" as part of my DESTRESS Protocol™ for getting well, losing weight, and feeling alive again.

But for now, let's focus on what we need to be aware as far as toxic food choices, so that we can make the best choices possible when we're shopping for food or eating out.

GMOS

GMO foods are a man-made laboratory creation intended to withstand high levels of pesticide spray.

To create some GMO foods, heavy metals and viruses must be used to change the genetic material of that original food to manufacture a new man-made one. Literally, GMO foods are "Frankenstein creations" made in a lab by inserting new genes into the DNA of current food crops or even fish.

These newly engineered foods contain no additional health benefits, but do possess the ability to harm you as a by-product of the heavy spraying used in conjunction with growing them.

Additional research is being done right now on their connection to low fertility, gut dysfunction, autoimmune diseases, autism, birth defects and other hormone related maladies.

What we do know right now is that in clinical studies, GMO soy fed to pregnant female rats leads to birth defects, low birth weight, and a high likelihood that their babies won't survive (increased risk of infant mortality).[18]

Those next generation babies were also found to be smaller and more infertile. The male rats fed GMO soy had increased testicular abnormalities and altered sperm.

Please also keep in mind that no outside long-term testing has been done on GMO foods yet – And the testing that is done is by the GMO manufacturer themselves.

This whole system is eerily similar to pharmaceutical drug testing. This means that the same people that produce the profit-driven substance are the same ones that get to test it. To me, something seems wrong with that picture…

I urge you to do your very best to avoid GMO foods. I believe more long-term and 3rd party GMO testing must be done to ensure our safety as well as our children's.

Furthermore, the main reason GMOs have been created is to allow for heavy crop spraying of pesticides, which, as you are about to learn, are potent cancer-causing chemicals on their own.

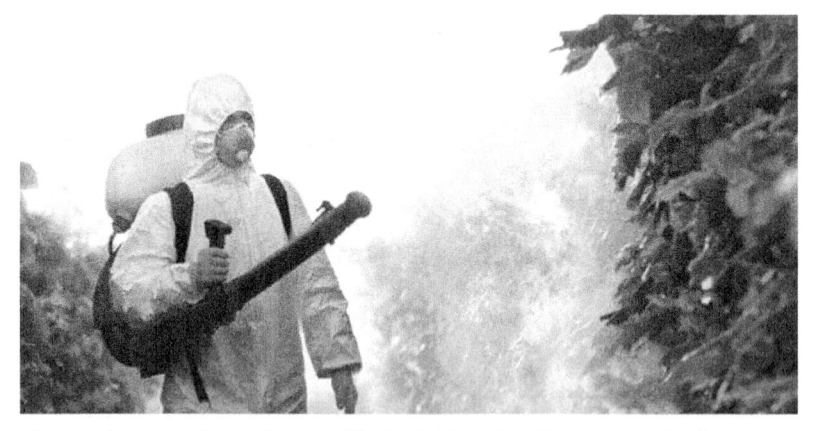

(This is what your fruits & vegetables look like when being sprayed. If the spray is so toxic that a HAZMAT suit needs to be worn, how is it deemed safe to eat?)

Here are the top GMO foods to avoid:

- Beets & Beet Sugar (95%)
- Canola Oil (93%)
- Cottonseed Oil (93%)
- Soy (93%)
- Corn (86%)
- Hawaiian Papaya (80%)
- Other GMOs include alfalfa, zucchini, squash, flax, GM salmon

Please also keep in mind that the by-products of GMOs must also be watched out for. These include all corn syrups, GMO sweeteners, lecithin's from soy, and vegetable oils/butter.

Plus, most farm animals you consume as meat and dairy, have been fed GMO soy, corn, and flax as part of their feed (unless otherwise stated as grass-fed, pasture raised, or organic).

HORMONES

Right now, the majority of the meat you're buying has been pumped full of steroids, estrogens, and growth hormones in order to stimulate the production of more muscle tissue (meat) and milk production.

The FDA has been allowing this since at least the 1950s, and in the 1990s many governments allowed for the use of recombinant bovine somatotropin (rBST) and recombinant bovine growth hormones (rBGH).

The good news is that countries in the European Union, Canada, Australia, Japan, New Zealand and Israel have been slowly banning these substances. We can only hope the U.S. will follow.

One of the reasons why these hormones are such a lightning rod for debate is that studies have found that milk from rBGH has 10x the amount of growth hormones (IGF-1) as regular milk.

And it is IGF-1 that the American Cancer Society and other groups have linked to prostate, colon, and other types of cancer.[19]

The larger amounts of hormones present in meat and dairy go well beyond implications for cancer. We are now seeing young girls beginning puberty at much younger ages today, with some girls beginning menstrual cycles under 10 years old.

A young girl's physiology and psychology is simply not biologically programmed to have the ability to carry a baby in a child's body.

In addition to the issues mentioned above, the meat industry uses a host of chemicals to "treat" the meat before it makes its way to stores and restaurants. Again, in order for me to not make this a 700-page encyclopedia to read and review, I urge you to look into the radiation and spraying of meat before it ever makes it to your table.

You can also consider the fact that sausage and ground beef often come from thousands of cattle (not one animal) and contain hooves, bone, anus meat and parts the animal's brain.

This is often why meat contamination is so high. And if you have the interest, check out how over 50% of all antibiotics are being used on farm animals to keep them from dying due to the unnatural and deplorable diet they're fed…

Later we'll discuss how you can easily find single-source, hormone-free meat, eggs, and dairy locally, if you decide to keep animal products as a part of your nutrition plan.

PRESERVATIVES

Food preservatives are added to meat and other products to prevent discoloration and rotting, as well as to extend shelf-life.

Preservatives are often hidden on labels, but when they do show up they may be called sulfites, nitrates, MSG, sodium benzoate, propyl gallate, aspartame, butylated hydroxytoluene (BHT), and phosphoric acid.

Food preservatives have been linked to:

- Cancers in lab animals
- Asthma and allergic reactions associated with chemicals, such as sulfites and nitrites (which prevent discoloration in meats and are considered one of the worst food additives ever created for human health)
- Bowel symptoms, such as nausea and diarrhea, which could be part of an allergic reaction
- Pre-term, premature births (artificial sweeteners)
- Hyperactivity and attention deficit disorder in children
- Human resistance to antibiotics because of use in food animals
- Headaches from substances such as monosodium glutamate (MSG)
- Increased risk of heart disease from an accumulation of phosphates in the body
- Risk of weight gain from added sugars and sweeteners, hormones, or substances that interfere with hormone regulation
- Neurological problems, like those from aspartame consumption.[20]

I'd also like to bring to your attention the fact that food dyes are placed in many beverages to give them color. Children's "treats" and candies often have these dyes as well, which are given fun names like Yellow #5 and Yellow# 6, and Red #40. (They are easy to spot since under the ingredients, there will be the name of a color, plus a number after it.)

Believe it or not, these colorful dyes are literally paint with all the toxins that come along with this man-made substance. The only reason these synthetic, cheaply-made chemicals are in your foods and beverages is to give them more "color" and market appeal.

In my practice, I see numerous childhood (and adult) learning and behavioral issues directly correlated to preservatives and food dyes.

One of the first things I do is remove those specific chemicals from their diet. I learned many years ago that this alone can make a huge difference in positive changes in mood and cognitive ability within just a few weeks of removal.

Lastly, I have also seen people suffering from psoriasis, eczema, and other skin issues see remarkable improvement once offending foods and preservatives were removed from their nutrition plan.

ARTIFICIAL SWEETENERS

Artificial sweeteners were developed to be sugar-free and to create low calorie lines of food for dieters and diabetics. They also allow food to be even sweeter to the taste than real, actual sugar.

But like most "foods" created in a lab, the science experiment went wrong and was only found out years later to be causing health concerns. Now we know artificial sweeteners can cause obesity, mood disorders, learning disabilities, neurological dysfunction, cancer, migraines, and cardiovascular disease.[21]

The most common artificial sweeteners go by these names:

- Aspartame
- Acesulfame K (potassium)
- Dulcin
- Equal
- Neotame
- NutraSweet
- Nutrinova
- Phenlalanine
- Saccharin
- Sucralose/Splenda
- Sweet 'N Low

Keep in mind, these sweeteners were made in a lab and are *not* real foods.

For example, Splenda® became popular awhile back and the public never knew that one of the ways this artificial sweetener is made is by replacing an existing molecule with chlorine.

Yes, that's the same chemical used in pool water.

The problem is chlorine effects your hormones, wipes out good bacteria in your gut, and the *Center for Science and Public Interest* placed Splenda® in its "caution category" in 2014 after studies showed it may cause leukemia.[22]

And then there are sugar alcohols like sorbitol and xylitol that have made their way into the marketplace. Some of the products that contain this substance include protein powders, energy bars, and snacks.

The issue with these pseudo-sugars that I see in my practice is that they cause serious gut issues in susceptible individuals. Bloating, gas, nausea, and diarrhea are not uncommon with consuming these types of sweeteners.

For more information on artificial sweeteners, please see my Cabral Concept podcast on this topic:
http://StephenCabral.com/284

Our food system is broken and there aren't enough people talking about it. It's certainly not taught in school and there's no way these companies are going to tell you what's really going into the fake food they pawn off as the real thing.

It's up to us to change the way we eat and view our food. The next Toxic Enemy on the list goes deeper into why GMOs and hormones may not even be the worst thing Big Pharma and Big Food is doing to our food supply…

Toxic Enemy #3
Pesticides & DDT

"Children who live in homes where their parents use pesticides [on the lawn] are twice as likely to develop brain cancer…"

- Agency for Toxic Substances and Disease Registry

I would like to believe that all these harmful synthetic substances were created with the benevolent intention to solve a problem.

However, like most man-made experiments released into our environment, what we often find (usually not until years later) is that these chemicals come along with some deadly side effects.

In the case of pesticides, we're now seeing horrific environmental and human consequences. Pesticides include herbicides that kill weeds, fungicides that kill fungus, insecticides that kill insects, and rodenticides that kill rodents.

Pesticides are essentially a nervous system poison that are used to deter bugs from eating the crops. These are highly poisonous bug sprays that have been dumped on our food supply to keep it from getting eaten by "pests."

While that sounds like a good idea, the downside is that we're swallowing bug spray every time we take a bite of a fruit, vegetable, or grain where it can't be washed off. And that's assuming that they can be completely washed off…

How does one ever wash off a raspberry's tender skin? How could the pesticide not penetrate the skin?

Glyphosates in pesticides like *Roundup* and other weed killers such as 2,4-D (Dichlorophenoxyacetic acid) are also known cancer causing agents.

And with continued use and sale, a strong causal link is being conclusively drawn between glyphosates and leukemia, non-Hodgkin's lymphoma, brain, bone, breast, ovarian, prostate, testicular and liver cancers.[23]

LONG-TERM DAMAGE

The information about pesticides isn't new.

We just aren't doing anything about it. Crops must be protected so they can be sold. We've known for over 20 years that 21 commonly used toxic pesticides cause birth defects.

These pesticides often show up in fetal cord blood, already poisoning the bodies and lives of our newborn children.

They are being exposed to cancer-causing chemicals before they're even out of the womb. Pesticide exposure in utero and in childhood has also been shown to cause ADD and ADHD due to the frontal lobe damage in the brain and destruction of neurotransmitters.[24]

And these pesticides don't just disappear once we stop using them. They can continue to poison our soil, water, and air for many years. A substance called DDT that has been linked to reproductive issues, male infertility, and nervous system damage is still being found in our food supply and dairy nearly 40 years after it was banned.

And according to one study conducted by the Center for Disease control, 99% of all people tested had byproducts of DDT (DDE) in their blood.[25]

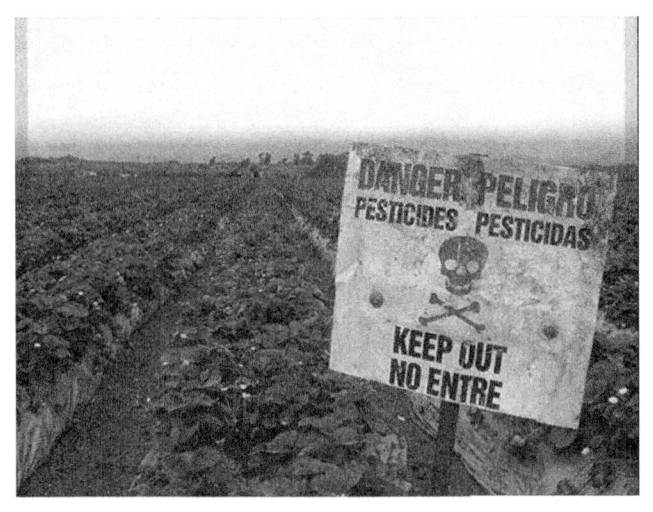

(Should your food in the grocery store also have a "skull and cross bones" sign on like it does out in the fields telling us to keep away?)

As bad as all those linked illnesses listed above are, they're only a fraction of what these chemicals can do to the human body.

The problem is that their prevalent use has now caused a domino effect of conditions, all acting as precursors to nervous system disorders, reproductive problems, learning disabilities in children, birth defects, autoimmune issues, mystery illnesses, and brain deterioration.

WE MUST STOP EATING BUG SPRAY

The reason for this is that the bug spray on our food overloads our liver and impairs our body's ability to detoxify.

This allows the chemicals to float freely around the blood stream and act as free radicals, which poison our cells.

The antibiotic effects of the bug spray also wipes out a lot of the good bacteria in our gut, causing a slow weakening of our gut wall and destroying our immunity along with it.

This is why that even if you believe in GMOs, it's hard to justify their long-term health benefits when they are some of the most heavily sprayed crops in the world.

Please keep in mind these same high-pesticide crops are also then fed to the animals you may be consuming as meat or dairy.

And, the water run-off from the pesticide sprayed crops then flows into our soil and drinking water supply.

DO PESTICIDES CAUSE CANCER?

Another startling fact is that a number of studies by the National Cancer Institute found that American farmers had far increased incidences of leukemia, Hodgkin's disease, non-Hodgkin's lymphoma, and many other forms of cancer.[26]

This is also not an issue specific to the United States. Overseas, as crop spraying has increased, the amount of cancer and reproductive disorders has risen.[27]

If that wasn't enough, the peer-reviewed journal IMCJ (Integrative Medicine: A Clinician's Journal) published an article in the February/March 2017 issue showing a direct correlation between the herbicide glyphosate found in products such as *Roundup*® and many other commercial herbicides (weed killers) and the presence of autism.[28]

Keep in mind, these are the same poisons that are allowed to be sprayed on all conventional food, GMO crops, and in people's backyards. It's literally a systemic problem that infiltrates every aspect of our world.

When you couple this with the statistic that lab researchers need just one pesticide to create cancer in lab rats, you can see why more people than ever are getting cancer today. This is a horrifying fact and one that too few people are talking about. Why is it that we're desperately searching for the "cure to cancer" and other diseases when we know exactly how it can be created?

This toxic threat of pesticides can become very technical, but what's most important to keep in mind is that what you put into your mouth most likely has more of an effect on your health than anything else in your life.

WHAT CAN WE DO?

Because of this, I urge you to choose organic whenever possible, and if you have the ability to shop at local farmer's markets, do so. It is at these local markets that you can speak with your city or state's farmers and see how they grow their food.

In the coming DESTRESS Protocol ™, you will discover the 12 foods never to eat grown conventionally, and the 15 that are "acceptable" to eat non-organic if you chose to.

The bottom line is that unless we consider alternative methods of growing our food, I fear we may be headed further down a path of increased cancer, brain atrophy, and genetic mutations within our DNA that will effect generations to come…

Before we move on to our next toxic enemy, I'd like to make you aware of another way in which chemicals like pesticides can make you sick.

We're hardly ever told that the chemicals they spray on golf courses, parks, or your grass can be toxic to your system.

Often, we stare at beautiful green grass in awe, but we fail to recognize that lush color comes at a severe cost.

Did you know that in just the last 10 years, a study was published by the Agency for Toxic Substance and Disease Registry showing that children who live in homes where their parents use pesticides [on the lawn] are twice as likely to develop brain cancer versus those that live in residences in which no pesticides are used?[29]

THE RESEARCH IS IRREFUTABLE

And right now, the back and forth arguments are simply based upon exposure, dosage, genetic predisposition, and the length of exposure time needed before one gets sick from the side effects of pesticides.

The good news is that you can use specific scientifically formulated detoxification protocols to remove these harmful pesticides from your body, and if you're so inclined, you can even test your current levels using an at-home urine based test.

The all-natural foods and products explained in the DESTRESS Protocol™ will help you lower or eliminate your toxic load. Remember, we need to be even more diligent nowadays about staying healthy in an unhealthy world!

Up next, I want to share with you why the water you're drinking may not be as "pure" as you've been led to believe…

Toxic Enemy #4
Tap Water

"The average 10-minute shower is the equivalent to drinking 20 gallons of tap water."

- Dr. Shulze, *Detox Special Report*, April 2013

First off, I want to say that I am grateful that we no longer live in an era where we have to be afraid of getting cholera, a parasite, or dysentery every time we drink water.

It's nice to know that many of the illnesses caused from impure drinking water have been removed and, in a pinch, we can turn on a faucet almost anywhere in the world and out comes "drinkable" water.

The problem is that the infectious pathogens formerly in our water have been replaced by a new generation of toxins. These toxins are just as deadly, but their effects, like most man-made chemicals, poison you slowly.

CHLORINE

Chlorine does help eliminate bacteria from your water, and it works exceptionally well.

It's also why it's used in public pools as a disinfectant.

However, the same powerful bacteria-fighting properties that make it great to clean your water also allow it to kill much of the good bacteria in your gut.

This means that every glass of tap water you drink, you're potentially wiping out your good gut probiotics from chlorine's antibiotic effects.

In the long run this can lead to a weakened immune system, leaky gut, and a host of chronic illnesses.

Chlorine is also now being linked to low thyroid conditions, since iodine becomes depleted as your body is exposed to this chemical from tap water, pools, and your daily shower.

The other major issue with chlorine is that it becomes a vapor as the hot water evaporates out of your shower, steam room, or bathtub. Believe it or not, chlorine was actually used as a chemical weapon in this very way during World War 1.

As a gas vapor, chlorine is more dangerous, since the chlorine can then enter directly into your bloodstream via your lungs. This type of gaseous exposure can cause permanent pulmonary damage, directly affecting your breathing.

FLUORIDE

In 1914, fluoride was added to toothpaste to try to help prevent cavities. Later, in 1962, the Department of Health and Human Services (DHHS) suggested that public tap water contain between 0.7 and 1.2 mgs. of fluoride per liter.

This was due to the now controversial belief that fluoride is more effective than unfluoridated toothpaste at preventing tooth decay.

However, studies in European countries that do not add fluoride to their water show no increase in cavities versus their counterparts.[30]

The one thing we do know is that fluoride is a confirmed poison.

As of 2017, the US Government has retracted their earlier recommendations and warns that the upper limit of fluoride added to tap water should be no more than 0.7mg per liter.

Also, keep in mind that the #1 call that the American Association of Poison Control Centers receives on a daily basis is from parents of sick children that have eaten toothpaste.

The acute-term ingestion of even just 4mg/l of fluoride in water will cause death, but it is through the slow poisoning of our bodies by chemicals such as fluoride that leads to what we classify today as dis-ease.

For example, tap water and fluoridated toothpaste consumption has been shown to correlate with these health conditions:

- low thyroid
- brittle bones
- weakened digestion
- hormone dysfunction
- GERD, acid reflux
- eczema, psoriasis
- fertility issues
- calcification of pineal gland
- lowering of IQ in children
- ADD, ADHD [31]
- autism[32]
- mental health disorders
- arthritis

YOUR THYROID ON FLUORIDE

I wish I could say that this was new information, but it's been known since the 1930's that fluoride affects thyroid function. German and Austrian doctors used to bathe patients with overactive thyroid disorders in tubs containing fluoridated water.

They knew even back then that fluoride lowers thyroid function and now we can scientifically prove why.

Both iodine and fluoride are chemical compounds called halogens. Your body uses iodine to nourish your thyroid, which in turn allows it to function normally. Fluoride can be taken up by your thyroid gland instead, thus blocking the need for iodine.

However, it gets worse. Fluoride is actually toxic to thyroid cells and kills them.

I wish I could say that it took a lot of fluoride to cause this effect, but the toxic effect of fluoride on the thyroid is the same level as that of the cutoff level of fluoride in tap water (.33mg/l).

FROM THE TOILET TO YOUR TAP

Mary Buzby of Merck Pharmaceuticals has stated, *"There's no doubt about it, pharmaceuticals are being detected in the environment and there is a genuine concern that these compounds, in the small concentrations they're at, could be causing impacts to human health or to the aquatic organisms."*

Before we move on to our next toxic enemy, I need to make you aware of one other harmful pollutant coming out of your faucet.

It's been a quiet concern of smaller consumer protection groups since the early 1990's, but the Associated Press, Natural Resources Defense Council, and other news organizations have blown the whistle recently on the fact that pharmaceutical drugs have been found in your tap water for decades.

A recent investigation revealed that all municipal water supplies tested contain some amount of pharmaceutical drugs. The most common drugs found are the hormones in birth control pills, blood thinners, blood pressure meds, antidepressants, mood stabilizers, and antibiotics.[34]

Although we're told by the Environmental Protection Agency (EPA) that the levels of these drugs are "safe" to consume, this thinking is somewhat shortsighted, to say the least.

What they mean is that these smaller quantities of pharmaceuticals won't cause immediate harm, but again we're talking about cumulative effects here – years and decades of daily exposure, which adds up over time.

Plus, children are far more susceptible to the affects of all toxins due to their less mature detoxification abilities and developing bodies and minds.

By now you may be asking yourself how is it possible for drugs to end up in my tap water? It's a great question and the truth is that many people flush their drugs down the toilet. And, the residual remains of metabolized drugs come out in a person's urine or stool. This means that the drugs a person takes or throws out in the toilet eventually makes into your family's drinking water.

Your next question may then be, "I thought my drinking water came from a natural spring or reservoir?"

A few years back I thought the same thing. Unfortunately, it's far from the truth. The reality is that more and more drinking water is actually just recycled sewage water.

Yes, you heard that right.

Your toilet waste water goes to a treatment plant where it is "cleaned" and then either dispersed into our oceans or funneled back into your home tap water. *(As a side note, you can also research more about how our fish are literally consuming the same pharmaceutical drugs we are now.)*

Cities like San Diego, are now drinking 85% "recycled" water, which they import from treatment facilities out of state. Drinking fresh spring water from pristine reservoirs seems to be becoming a thing of the past...[35]

Please keep in mind that bottled water isn't much better since 25% of manufacturers simply just bottle tap water, they then resell to you for over $1 a bottle.

As always, you do have a choice and you can protect yourself and your family with simple measures. I'll explain these options in depth during the DESTRESS Protocol ™.

Now that you know how the chemicals in tap water can account for many of the health issues you or your loved ones may be dealing with, I'd like to switch gears and move away from our focus on food and beverages. Our next Top 10 Toxic Enemy concerns a "chemical" we are producing all on our own...

Toxic Enemy #5
Stress

> *"39% of people report overeating or eating unhealthy foods due to stress."*
>
> - AMERICAN PSYCHOLOGICAL ASSOCIATION

It's hard for most of us to believe that stress could be the underlying root cause of 90% of all disease in the world…

After all, stress is a normal part of life, right?

The answer to that is not so straightforward.

Although stress is a completely normal human response in both mind and body, the way in which we now respond to stress on a physical, mental, and emotional level in the 21st century is completely abnormal.

Stress is meant to be a finite occurrence that has both a beginning and an end.

However, our daily stresses have been compounded in this technological age with limitless stimulation, activities, work, family obligations, and a seemingly frantic drive to keep up with everything. This keeps us running on the proverbial hamster wheel in perpetual motion with no finish line in sight…

We hope to slow down, we tell ourselves, when we retire. But many of the stressors in our daily environment never stop coming and have little to do with work anymore.

The problem is that for many people that day of relief from stress never comes. Or if it does, it's too late. Many traumas, stresses, and physical and emotional setbacks have been suffered throughout the previous decades and have now accumulated and taken their toll.

While much of this work/life/relationship stress can be mitigated using lifestyle changes like the *DESTRESS Protocol*™, what isn't very well known is that stress is more than just our emotional response to outside forces.

THE XENOBIOTIC INVASION

There is something called xenostressors, which literally means "outside stressors".

These xenostressors are further classified as xenobiotics, which means "chemicals foreign to the body."

These toxic enemies are the heavy metals, pesticides, electromagnetic waves, exhaust fumes, pollution, all the toxins in our environment, that make their way into our body from our food, water, and air supply. They then cause a predictable, although unfavorable, reaction in our body, as our body attempts to detoxify them but ultimately fails.

Remember, these xenobiotics are poisonous to the body and will kill the body (or cause dis-ease) if the body does not detoxify and clean them out fast enough.

These external stressors are a major source of internal stress on the body now. After all, it is literally life or death as far as your body is concerned.

So between both emotional stress and outside toxins, we are unwittingly throwing our bodies (and mind) into what's called the fight or flight reaction. And it's constant.

I will explain this in more detail, but for now here is a short summary of what happens and why this is so important to understand.

When your brain receives a signal that a toxin has entered the body, a part of the brain stem called the Locus Coeruleus lights up like a Christmas Tree. It is at this point that norepinephrine is released, which puts your body in an excited and stimulated state.

This norepinephrine then triggers the amygdala portion of your brain, which relates to feelings of anxiety, fear, panic, and anger/ rage.

During this cascade, the hypothalamus and pituitary gland become activated and release additional stress hormones called CRH and ACTH, which cause our adrenal glands to secrete adrenaline from the adrenal medulla and cortisol from the adrenal cortex.

The Stress Reaction Aerobics

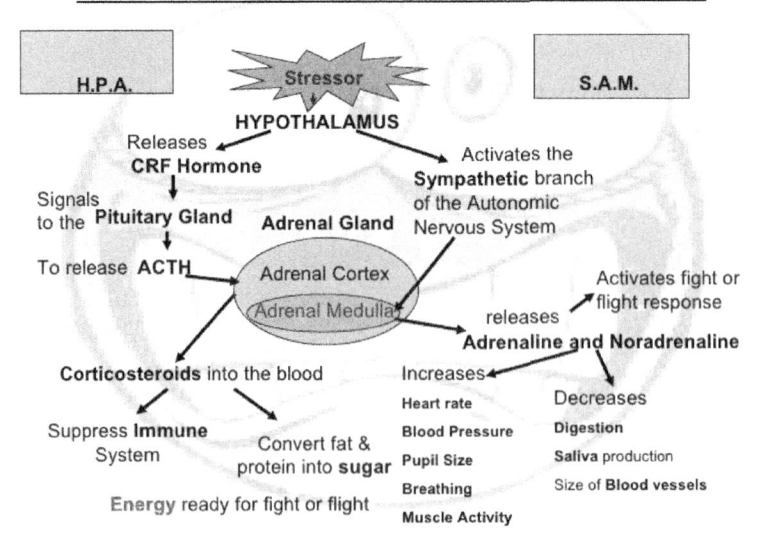

H.P.A. — Stressor → **HYPOTHALAMUS** — **S.A.M.**

Releases **CRF Hormone**
Signals to the **Pituitary Gland**
To release **ACTH**
→ Adrenal Cortex / Adrenal Medulla (Adrenal Gland)

Activates the **Sympathetic** branch of the Autonomic Nervous System
releases **Adrenaline and Noradrenaline**
Activates fight or flight response

Corticosteroids into the blood
Suppress **Immune** System
Convert fat & protein into **sugar**
Energy ready for fight or flight

Increases:
Heart rate
Blood Pressure
Pupil Size
Breathing
Muscle Activity

Decreases:
Digestion
Saliva production
Size of Blood vessels

(The above graphic shows how stress affects our entire body and mind.)

All of this may seem like very complex endocrinology, but what's essential to understand is that stress is literally one of the most fundamental cornerstones of health that must be managed and healed in order for anyone to become well.

You don't need complex biochemistry in order to understand intuitively that when your body and mind are stressed – whether that stress arises from trauma, a violent relationship, or from the toxic stress of being exposed to the over 77,000 man-made chemicals in the environment, your body feels that it is under attack.

Over time, this constant bombardment of internal and external stressors eventually wears the body down, burns out the central nervous system, and keeps us locked into a pattern of sympathetic nervous system stress (fight or flight).

The problem is that repair, recovery, and rejuvenation do not take place until we can relax. And we can't relax while we're locked in a constant fight or flight state.

So until we can move our body into the healing state of the parasympathetic nervous system, we cannot fully recover our body, mind, or vitality.

This is a crucial piece to the puzzle, since it doesn't matter what health or weight issue you're dealing with, if your body is under stress it simply cannot heal.

If you can't make a shift from the sympathetic nervous system of stress to the parasympathetic relaxed state you will always be fighting an uphill battle to get well.

Now are you beginning to see how a life filled with both internal emotional stress and outside toxicity can combine to cause an over-stimulated dis-ease state?

It's also one of the main reasons why therapy alone may not work for many people with anxiety, panic attacks, OCD, depression or other mood disorders. Until you remove the REAL causes, no amount of willpower, medication, or therapy can help you achieve wellness.

The good news is that by combining the best of the ancient healing secrets of the East with the state-of-the-art Naturopathic and Functional Medicine science, you can re-regulate the stress hormone pathways.

This will then allow you to get well, lose the weight, and feel alive again!

I share the exact strategies I use in my practice for overcoming stress in all forms in the "Stress" chapter of the DESTRESS Protocol ™.

As we now move onto Toxic Enemy #6, we're going to review (maybe for the first time) how a more recent "invisible" toxin all around us is effecting our nervous system, brain, DNA, and immunity.

Toxic Enemy #6
Electrosmog

"Nervous system disorders, fatigue, poor sleep, Leukemia in children, breast cancer or cancer clusters have been linked to high exposure to EMFs."

- NATIONAL CANCER INSTITUTE

It's invisible to the eye, yet it is one of the most disturbing occurrences going on all around us. It's called "electrosmog" and it refers to the electromagnetic frequencies (EMFs) and waves that are moving through our living matrix.[36,37,38]

Our bodies are literally 99.9% energy and because of this, we are subject to the same electromagnetic disturbances in our energy.

This means that the cell phones, computers, Wi-Fi modems, cell towers, and any electronic equipment can damage the cell to cell communication within our body.

This can then lead to immune dysfunction, mitochondrial energy fatigue, increased fight or flight, gut bacterial disturbances, and even cancer.

But since this new threat is invisible and most of us can't directly feel its immediate effect, we dismiss it like most other toxins we're exposed to at a low level.

The problem, like with these other Top 10 Toxins, is that the day in and day out exposure continues to accumulate and eventually wears down our disease-fighting defense mechanisms.

ELECTROMAGNETIC HYPERSENSITIVITY (EHS)

Current science does also recognize a syndrome called *electromagnetic hypersensitivity*. The problem is that it's a diagnosis typically reserved for those that have been exposed to a massive dose of radiation.

Thousands of cases are being reported by regular people who are experiencing symptoms of fatigue, illness, anxiety, depression, hopelessness, irregular heartbeat, skin rashes, swollen lymph nodes and other physical and mental abnormalities.

It appears that when a susceptible individual is exposed to multiple electronic machines such as microwaves, alarm clocks, cell phones, and modems, the EMF waves are disturbing their cellular balance.

It's important to note that many of these cases come from people with metal already inside their body, such as "silver" amalgam dental work fillings, joint replacements, metal IUDs, plates, screws, heavy metal cellular build up, etc. It appears that the different metals are possibly acting as beacons that conduct electrical currents in the body.

In many cases, using a heavy metal detox, grounding techniques, and eliminating as many EMF sources as possible help symptoms to subside.

Although medical science has yet to be able to verify EHS, if you currently suffer from what could be electrosmog poisoning, it's important to use an EMF detector to see what sources in your home or office are transmitting the strongest frequencies.

It may also be worth considering having any heavy metal in your body that's able to be taken out (replacing dental fillings, etc.) removed by a professional.

CELL PHONE STUDY

We all know that cell phones are a fixture in our life. But did you know that the long-term effects of cell phone use have been shown to cause brain tumors?[39]

Cell phones in fact, have been found to cause tumors on the breasts of women who keep them in their bras.[40]

The scariest part is that the tumors are happening at a much faster rate in children. In general, a child's body is far more susceptible to these EMFs and radiation than a full-grown adult.

As I said before, I don't think anyone of us is going to get rid of our cell phone anytime soon, but you do need to be aware of its dangers and try to limit its use as much as possible.

The good news is that by simply using a wired headset while talking on your phone you can dramatically reduce the amount of radiation to your brain. *(Wireless Bluetooth headsets increase EMF exposure.)*

Also, for children, it is best that you turn their cell phones, iPad, tablets, etc. to "airplane" mode while in use. This will turn off the Wi-Fi signal and reduce EMF exposure to their brain and organs whenever they place an electronic device on their laps.

"SMART" METERS

I'd also be remiss if I didn't make you aware of the new biggest EMF threat to our health.

They're called, "Smart Meters," and you may already have one attached to your home. These meters are essentially boxes that measure your electricity use and then beam that data back to your local electricity provider.

All of this sounds well and good and just another amazing technological advancement, so that your meter doesn't have to be read manually, but it does come at a cost.

The cost, of course, is your health and the effects are potentially even more damaging to children and pets who are smaller and more susceptible.

Although I'll be giving you tips, tricks, strategies, and much more in my DESTESS Protocol™, I want to make you aware that you can deny a smart meter from being added to your home.

And, if you already do have one attached to your house, you can mitigate many of its effects by covering it with an EMF mat.

(All RBE recommendations and resources are available all in one place at: StephenCabral.com/rbe)

THE FUTURE

Artificial intelligence, virtual reality, scanners, and additional smart shopping and home devices are only going to increase with each coming year.

It is the future and there is no stopping it…

It's going to be very interesting to see how we combat this level of electrosmog when every store, room in our home, and means of transportation are bombarding us with notifications and wrapping us in digital wave technology.

Right now our best bet is to reduce exposure whenever possible.

For example, modems can also be switched off at night, and computers, tablets, and cell phones can be powered down or at least kept out of your bedroom.

My highest recommendation is to at least keep your bedroom EMF-free while you sleep. This gives you 8 hours of true EMF detoxification and cellular healing.

I'll be sharing more tips to stay EMF-safe, but for now let's look at Toxic Enemy #7. This is the one that many of us need to consider most since we spend the majority of time at work or in our homes…

Toxic Enemy #7
Home Sick

> *"Americans spend 90% of their time indoors. Most people take in 126 toxins every day before ever leaving the house and it takes just 26 seconds for these chemicals to get into your blood stream…"*
>
> - OrthoMolecular Products Inc., March, 2014

In 1984, the World Health Organization stated that approximately 1/3rd of all new buildings could be causing acute illness.

That was over 30 years ago . . .

The use of synthetic materials has only increased and with it so too has the increase in environmental toxins.

The issue with home and office buildings is that they are built so well that the indoor toxins can't escape! This means that the air you breathe is literally infected with toxins you can't see, but you most certainly are breathing them in.

The situation has gotten so bad that we now have two names to describe how people are being affected by these toxins: *sick building syndrome* and *sick home syndrome*.

SICK BUILDING SYNDROME

The first one called, "Sick Building Syndrome," refers mainly to office buildings where you may work or visit.

These structures usually contain multiple floors and often the chemicals that the business uses compound the already toxic carpets, insulation, and cleaning products used in the building.

Plus, office buildings are notorious for having poor air quality due to mold or bacteria build up in the HVAC venting systems.

SICK HOME SYNDROME

The 2nd toxic environment you are most definitely being exposed to is something called *Sick Home Syndrome*, or *Toxic Home Syndrome*.

This term became of increasing interest after it was reported that 15.3 million homes in the UK contain up to 900 chemicals in the air and have been causing an array of allergy, mood, skin, brain fog, watery eyes, and respiratory issues.[41]

One of the best signs to begin to understand if your office or home (or any building) is making you sick is to see if your symptoms subside when you leave and pick back up when you re-enter that space.

The other issue with home or office toxicity is that most people don't have an immediate reaction. Therefore, they don't notice what is going on in their body and it allows for the chemicals to build up from these exposures over time.

Then, weeks, months, or years later, they finally see the signs and symptoms that their body can no longer keep all the chemicals that need to be detoxed for the health of the system at bay.

It's at this point that the initial trigger has caused a deeper inflammatory and detox response from the body. Simply removing yourself from that environment will not be enough.

You can of course still heal, but your protocol will be now focused on healing the dis-ease symptoms, as well as changing your environment.

Toxic chemicals in your home and body

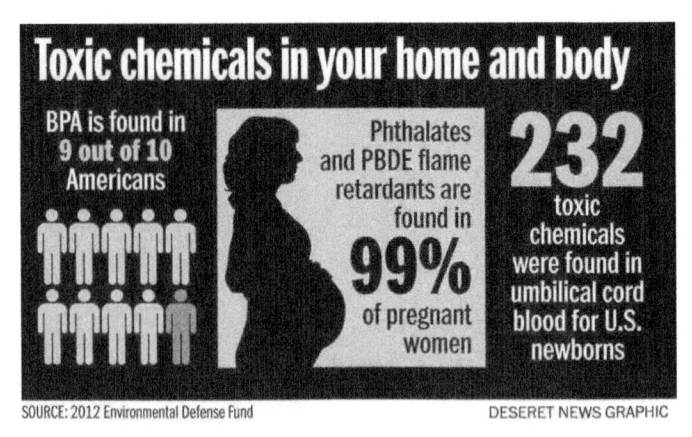

BPA is found in 9 out of 10 Americans

Phthalates and PBDE flame retardants are found in 99% of pregnant women

232 toxic chemicals were found in umbilical cord blood for U.S. newborns

SOURCE: 2012 Environmental Defense Fund   DESERET NEWS GRAPHIC

(As detailed above the toxicity threat is real and it affects everyone of us. Even those yet to be born – More on this specific topic to come later in this book.)

WHAT TO WATCH OUT FOR

Here are just a few of the invisible chemicals you may be exposed to in your home of office:

- Bathroom air fresheners
- Cleaning products
- Dryer sheets
- Synthetic perfumes and fragrances
- Lead paint
- Paint fumes
- Varnishes
- Urethanes on floor
- Vinyl's
- Polyurethane
- Synthetic insulation
- Smoke (cigarettes, candles, cooking, etc.)
- Paint fumes
- Mold spores
- Mildew

- Dust mites
- Synthetic carpet outgassing
- Pet dander & allergens
- Flame retardant particles
- Fabric outgassing
- Natural gas and carbon dioxide
- Construction materials
- Chlorine from bath & shower water vapors
- Lead or toxic paint
- Carbon monoxide
- Car garage solvents and fumes
- Oil and gas fumes

Please understand the chemicals listed above are a real threat to your health and safety.

Lead paint alone still causes approximately 1,000,000 children a year to have to go to the hospital due to poisoning It's not enough to just be aware of the dangers – we must act and do something about it.

I do understand that there may not be a lot you can do about your office work environment, but you can be aware of what to look for and raise any issues that you now see in your building.

Additionally, in the "Toxins" portion of the DESTRESS Protocol™, I will be sharing with you my recommendations for non-toxic home cleaning products and other items that will keep you and your family safe from these invisible chemicals.

SPECIAL NOTE

Some jobs are more toxic than others. For example, firefighters are exposed to higher levels of chemicals than the average person.

The reason for this is that they are literally running into buildings with burning plastic, asbestos, flame retardants, and other synthetic toxins, many of which have been proven to cause cancer.

It's also most likely the reason why firefighters have much higher levels of cancer.

Whether you're a firefighter, live secluded in the woods, or somewhere in between, I can assure you there is hope. Further in this book I will be sharing my Functional Medicine protocol for helping you to remove toxins from your cells, brain and blood.

This will allow you to reach a state of equilibrium, so that when new toxins come in, you are much better equipped to safely deal with and quickly eliminate them.

Now that we've reviewed the indoor air pollutants that can be taking their toll on your health, I'd like to share with you the specific products you may be placing on your skin daily that you don't even know are loaded with synthetic chemicals.

This is mandatory information we should all know!

Toxic Enemy #8
Skin Care Products

"The average woman uses 12 beauty or skin products a day that contain over 168 different (toxic) chemicals."

- Scott Faber, Environmental Working Group (EWG)

Did you know that you absorb up to 60% of what you place on your skin?

This includes the shampoos, conditioners, moisturizers, oils, hair styling products, lip balm, sunscreen, lipstick, and anything else you may apply topically.

All of these products add up quickly, which can cause hidden health triggers over time if the wrong products are being used.

COSMETIC CHEMICALS

Now that you know the average woman uses 12 beauty and skin care products that contain over 168 different chemicals, I want to share why this is a dangerous daily routine.[14]

I'd also like to add that the worst part is that many of these toxic chemicals aren't even required to be listed on the label. You see, the cosmetic industry isn't regulated the same way the food industry is regulated.

Technically, you can even label a skin care product "organic" even if it's not 100% organic. It's disturbing and deceitful to say the least…

The biggest problem of all, though, is that it's actually worse to place chemicals on your skin than it is to ingest them.

The reason is that when you eat pesticides or other toxins enter your saliva, then your natural enzymes, stomach acid, and bile at least get the opportunity to destroy some of these volatile compounds.

But when you place these same toxins directly on your skin, they get absorbed directly into your blood stream. It only takes 26 seconds for the absorption process to take place.

Sometimes the side effects of these cosmetic chemicals cause an immediate reaction that looks like an allergy, skin rash, headache, mood disturbance, brain fog, or fatigue.

However, for the most part, the chemicals just continue to compound on a daily basis and then eventually lead to cancer, fertility issues, birth defects, neurological disturbances, allergies, and auto-immune issues.

This is why it's so important that you do not take the "wait and see" approach.

Remember, these toxins accumulate over time and unless you're being mindful of cutting down on your exposure, you could very well be another victim of toxin overload.

For this reason, I recommend paying specific attention to all labels, not just food labels.

SHAMPOO
Average number of chemicals: 15

EYE SHADOW
Chemicals: 26

LIPSTICK
Chemicals: 33

BLUSH
Chemicals: 16

BODY LOTION
Chemicals: 32

FAKE TAN
Chemicals: 22

DEODORANT
Chemicals: 15

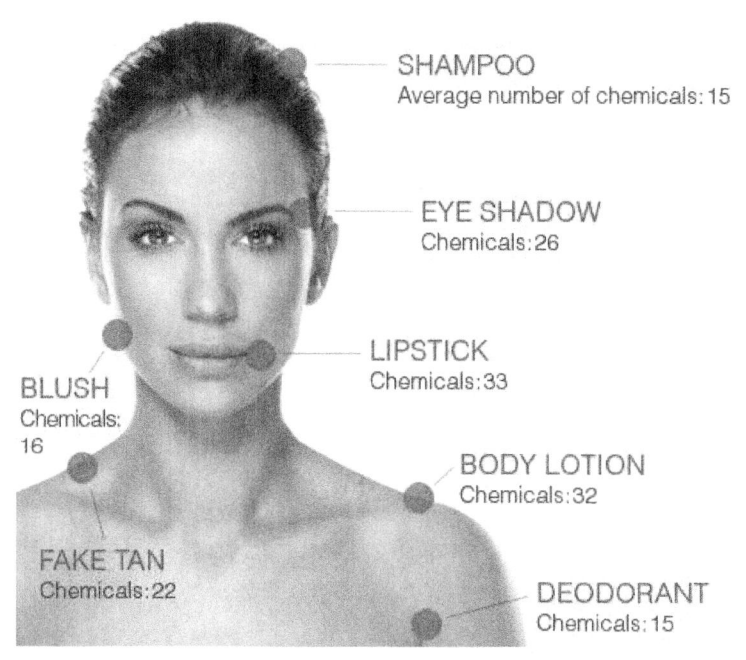

(It's unfortunate that companies aren't forced to place warning labels on their products even though we know many of these chemicals lead to disease, infertility, birth defects, and cancer.)

In terms of cosmetics, I've compiled a long list of specific and dangerous ingredients to look for below.

WHAT TO WATCH OUT FOR

Coal Tar: A known carcinogen banned in the European Union (EU) but still used in North America. Used in dry skin treatments, anti-lice and anti-dandruff shampoos, also listed as a color plus number. (i.e. FD&C Red No. 6.)

DEA/TEA/MEA: Suspected carcinogens used as emulsifiers and foaming agents for shampoos, body washes, soaps.

Ethoxylated surfactants and 1,4-dioxane: Never listed because it's a by-product made from adding carcinogenic ethylene oxide to make other chemicals less harsh. The Environmental Working Group (EWG) has found 1,4-dioxane in 57 percent of baby washes in the U.S. Avoid any ingredients containing the letters "eth."

Formaldehyde: Probable cancer causing carcinogen and irritant found in nail products, hair dye, fake eyelash adhesives, shampoos. Banned in the EU.

Fragrance/Perfume: A catchall for hidden chemicals, such as phthalates. Fragrance is connected to headaches, dizziness, asthma, and allergies.

Hydroquinone: Used for lightening skin. Banned in the UK, rated most toxic on the EWG's Skin Deep database, and linked to cancer and reproductive toxicity.

Lead: Known carcinogen found in lipstick and hair dye, but never listed because it's a contaminant, not an ingredient.

Mercury: Known allergen that impairs brain development. Found in mascara and some eye drops.

Mineral oil: By-product of petroleum that's used in baby oil, moisturizers, styling gels. It creates a film that impairs the skin's ability to release toxins.

Oxybenzone: Active ingredient in chemical sunscreens that accumulates in fatty tissues and is linked to allergies, hormone disruption (increases estrogen), cellular damage, low birth weight.

Parabens: Used as preservatives, found in many products. Linked to cancer, endocrine (hormone) disruption, reproductive toxicity.

Paraphenylenediamine (PPD): Used in hair products and dyes, but toxic to skin and immune system.

Phthalates: Plasticizers banned in the EU and California in children's toys, but present in many fragrances, perfumes, deodorants, lotions. Linked to endocrine hormone disruption, liver/kidney/lung damage, cancer.

Placental extract: Used in some skin and hair products- it is linked to endocrine hormone disruption.

Polyethylene glycol (PEG): Penetration enhancer used in many products, it's often contaminated with 1,4-dioxane and ethylene oxide, both known carcinogens.

Silicone-derived emollients: Used to make a product feel soft, these don't biodegrade, and prevent skin from breathing. Linked to tumor growth and skin irritation.

Sodium lauryl (ether) sulfate (SLS, SLES): A former industrial degreaser now used to make soap foamy, it's a toxin absorbed into the body and irritates skin.

Talc: Similar to asbestos in composition, it's found in baby powder, eye shadow, blush, dry shampoo and deodorant. Linked to ovarian cancer and respiratory problems.

Toluene: Known to disrupt the immune and endocrine systems, and negatively impact fetal development. It's used in nail and hair products. Often hidden under "fragrance."

Triclosan: Found in antibacterial products, hand sanitizers, and deodorants, it is linked to cancer and endocrine disruption.

(List credit: Dr. Gillian Deacon's Book, There's Lead in Your Lipstick, as quoted on TreeHugger.com)

I know the list above is a long one to continually cross-reference each time you purchase a product, so my initial recommendation is to look for organic, food-grade cosmetics, shampoos, etc., whenever possible. This means that you want to use products where you could literally eat what is inside the package.

Also try to shop at local or online retailers who already commit to non-toxic and organic skin, hair, and beauty care. This will help ensure that most of the products they carry already meet a much higher standard and do not contain a majority of the toxins listed above.

(And of course, at StephenCabral.com/rbe I'll continue to update the unbiased recommendations I use in my practice)

DAILY SUNSCREEN DANGERS

Although the FDA has directly stated, *"We are not aware of data demonstrating that sunscreen use alone helps prevent skin cancer,"* sunscreen has somehow become synonymous with lowering your chance of skin cancer.

The truth is sunscreen alone has not shown to lower your cancer risk, and most common brands may just increase it…

I know this is going to come as a shock, but the same sunscreen you've been told to wear daily to prevent skin cancer can actually cause it.

Yes, you read that right. The same sunscreen being touted as keeping away skin cancer can actually cause the same thing it's trying to prevent.

Here's why…

Over 70% of all sunscreens contain these chemicals below, which all have been verified to disrupt hormones (increase estrogen) and your immune system:

- Oxybenzone
- Avobenzone
- Octisalate
- Octocrylene
- Homosalate
- Octinoxate
- PABA esters
- Octisalate
- Homosalate
- Menthyl anthranilate
- Methylchloroisothiazolinone (MCI)
- Avobenzone
- Salicylates
- Digalloyl trioleate
- Cinnamates
- Benzophenoones (dioxybenzone, oxybenzone)
- Retinyl Palmitate[42]

The Center for Disease Control has now detected Oxybenzone in 96% of the population (children and adults) that they've tested.[43]

This means we have a population of people walking around unknowingly with chemicals in their bloodstream that cause allergies, mood disorders, inflammation, immune imbalance, low sperm count, and increases in estrogen.

All of which can then lead to cancer and speed up the growth of cancer already in the body.

WHAT ABOUT VITAMIN D?

Plus, using sunscreen all day lowers levels of vitamin D.

And low levels of vitamin D may lead to an increased likelihood of cancer cells proliferating and dozens of other diseases.

Plus, the whole idea that "it's only safe to get 15 minutes of sun" is not really true.

As an example, do you think someone with fair skin and someone with dark skin both need equal amounts of sun?

The answer is absolutely not.

Each individual needs an amount specific to his or her own physiology in order to produce and sulfate adequate vitamin D from the sun. Depending on the person, this may be 15-minutes or 5-hours.

This misinformation that there is a one-size-fits-all approach is one more media and corporate agenda trick to get us to fear the sun.

To be clear, I'm not advocating getting a sunburn or allowing your skin to turn "red" when outside.

You should never get burnt. Burning does damage your skin, inflames your immune system, and can cause further health issues. What I'm advocating is safe sun exposure to enhance immunity and detoxification, as well as prevent cancer.

This means you can remain in the sun uncovered for enough time to get a light pink hue on your skin. At this time, it is best to get out of the sun, cover up, or wear non-carcinogenic mineral (not chemical) sunscreen.

In the upcoming DESTRESS Protocol™, which offers the solution to getting and staying healthy in a toxic world, I will provide you with specific, safe, skincare recommendations for you and your family. Plus, I'll share an independent website that allows you to look up any product for yourself and find it's "toxic rating."

This next section on Toxic Enemy #9 is quite controversial, but needs to be said. It's the reason I believe many people can't get well, and it's making people a lot sicker.

It was also one of the main catalysts that caused me to become so sick at a young age…

Toxic Enemy #9
Pharmaceuticals

"Nearly 70 percent of Americans are on at least one prescription drug, and more than half take two…"

- The National Institute on Aging and the Mayo Clinic Center for the Science of Health Care Delivery[44]

Pharmaceuticals can be the most amazing life-saving interventions in the world. They can save your life.

The problem is that drugs are hardly ever needed for your average individual.

What I mean by that is there is absolutely no need to take a prescription drug unless your life is literally in danger—a situation where if you didn't take the drug, you would most likely die.

For every other situation and I mean literally all non-life saving conditions, natural medicine is the absolute best option.

The reason for this is that whenever you take a prescription drug (and yes, it is a drug), you are causing some other side effect inside your body.

Often, the long-term consequences of using drugs are far worse than the condition they were initially intended to treat.

Plus, pharmaceutical drugs used in chronic conditions, such as auto-immune diseases, are simply masking your symptoms. They literally do nothing to treat the underlying root cause of your condition which continues to fester under the surface.

This is the greater problem at work because while on the drug, you believe you are now well again, since your symptoms have disappeared.

It works, you think. I'm cured!

The unfortunate part is that in reality you are only getting worse. This is the reason why you see people with high cholesterol then get type 2 diabetes and high blood pressure.

The reason is that the hidden imbalance is still causing inflammation, and the sea of side effects then creates a tidal wave of more and more symptoms of dis-ease.

THE SIDE EFFECTS ARE REAL

Additionally, the drugs themselves have massive side effects that have been studied, researched, and proven to be detrimental to your long-term health.

For example, there are over 900 studies on just statin drugs alone.

This popular drug that more than 25% of the population over age 45 years old now takes has been scientifically proven to cause:

- Muscle weakness
- Muscle death
- Type 2 Diabetes
- Cardio myopathy (weak heart)

- Neurological issues
- Liver damage
- Acidosis
- Anemia
- Sexual dysfunction
- Cataracts
- Memory Loss[45,46]

Did you see how one of the side effects is a weakening of the heart?

This means that by taking a statin, you can still die of heart related issues even though you're lowering cholesterol and supposedly protecting your heart health!

To me and my Functional Medicine colleagues, this doesn't make any sense, especially since rebalancing cholesterol is one of the simplest fixes in natural medicine.

This same type of example holds true for high blood pressure, auto-immune disease, skin issues, migraines, fatigue, hormone imbalance, weight gain, and any other health condition you could think of.

Unless it's a congenital birth defect with non-repairable damage to an organ, there is simply no need to be on drugs. But this isn't what the pharmaceutical industry wants you to know.

They want you hooked on drugs like Prilosec (used to reduce acid reflux) that bring in billions of dollars alone from just that one pill.

But did you know that Prilosec, like many other drugs, has a warning that it should not to be used for more than 2 weeks?[47]

The reason is that this drug shuts down stomach acid production. You may think this is a good thing when you're suffering from an ulcer, GERD, or indigestion, but it's not.

People who take Prilosec or any PPI, severely limit their body's ability to digest food (you need stomach acid to break down protein!). This can then lead to parasites invading your intestines, malnourishment, osteoporosis from the poor absorption of calcium and other minerals, and IBS.

Now ask yourself, when was the last time you heard of anyone coming off Prilosec after just two weeks?

The answer is almost never.

Sadly, most doctors are not taught in medical school why someone would get acid reflux in the first place. And, if you're never taught why acid reflux would occur from a whole-body system perspective, how could you ever know what to look for and rebalance to help your patient?

The bottom line is that it's not your doctor's fault. It's a broken medical system that dictates a broken conventional medicine educational system...

THE SYSTEM IS BROKEN

This broken system then leads to an army of doctors that are specifically instructed to match up your current symptoms to a drug that they can prescribe, which is then covered by your health insurance.

It's the perfect business model:

- Drug companies pay professors to talk about specific drugs during class
- Medical school teaches future doctors to match drugs to symptoms
- Insurance companies pay for the drugs
- Drug companies get you hooked on their product
- The drug you take causes side effects, which then leads to additional drugs being prescribed to mask those symptoms
- Drug use causes life-long dependence on a monthly subscription plan that you pay for

Can you now see why the "healthcare" industry makes up 16% of the US economy?[48]

This is why drug companies have carte blanche and out-number congressman 2 to 1 with their lobbyist to make sure that laws are enacted to keep their profits soaring.

NO MORE BAND-AID APPROACHES

In my Functional Medicine practice I have honestly never seen a reason for someone to be on pharmaceutical drug for the rest of their life.

There are cases, but it is extremely rare and if you're on a drug right now, there's almost certainly a solution to wean you off that drug.

I believe this is an important distinction as well. I feel I'd be doing you a disservice to recommend that you just take yourself off any pharma drug you've been prescribed.

Remember, you can't pretend that you're not suffering from some type of imbalance. And until we correct that, you do have to be doing something.

This is why when I see someone in my practice on a cocktail of drugs, I don't have them wean off with their PCP until their symptoms subside by following a protocol just like the one you'll be getting in Part 4.

Although I could go on and on about the dangers and non-necessity of pharmaceuticals in chronic health conditions, I want to leave you with just one last note.

Even in what seems like the hardest to treat case, there is always a natural protocol that can be implemented to rebalance your body and treat the underlying root causes keeping you from optimum health and wellness.

You can get well!

In our final section on our Top 10 Toxic Enemies, we'll be dealing with the most under-rated cause for all diseases, inflammation, and weight gain. It is honestly the first place most people should be looking when trying to rebalance their body and mind…

Toxic Enemy #10
Gut Bugs

> *"Your gut health is critical to the health of your entire body. It's your first line of defense against cancer!"*
>
> - THE TRUTH ABOUT CANCER

It's not something most of us like to think about, but you harbor about 3-5 *pounds* of bacteria in your intestines.

And the amazing fact is that with over 100 trillion bacteria in your gut, there is actually more bacteria in your gut than there are cells in your entire body. Now that's a lot of bacteria!

The good news is that when your gut is balanced, bacteria helps manufacture vitamins, digest food properly, keeps your body lean, and your mind cheery.

The problem is that when the gut is imbalanced, everything silently suffers.

Outwardly though, you'll see symptoms like acne, anxiety, alcoholism, addiction, fatigue, weight gain, bloating, auto-immune issues, and cancer.

Inwardly, the root cause is gut dysbiosis (imbalanced bacterial terrain) and increased intestinal permeability (leaky gut).

This fact is no longer in dispute and gut dysbiosis or leaky gut has now been implicated in at least 90% of auto-immune diseases and many others.

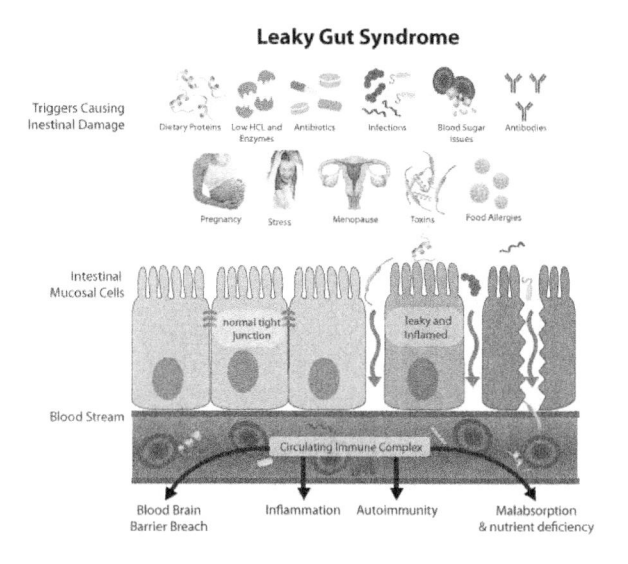

Leaky Gut Syndrome

("Leaky Gut" is no longer a "pseudo-science" as once believed. It is now at the center of almost all dis-eases within the body.)

The reason for this is that your gut associated lymphoid tissue (GALT), Peyer's patches, and other immune centers in and around your 28 feet of intestinal tract, represent up to 80% of your entire immune system.

Yes, you read that correctly – 80% of your immune system lies in your gut.

That means if you suffer from any health, weight gain, mood, or other disorder, it's essential that you heal your gut.

There may be other health matters to address as well, but if you aren't addressing the underlying issues with your digestive system and GALT, it will be challenging to ever fully recover.

WHAT TO WATCH OUT FOR

Some of the issues with your digestive tract that can hold you back from optimum health are:

- Candida, yeast, fungal overgrowth
- Bacterial overgrowth (SIBO)
- Parasites
- H. Pylori

Although bacteria and candida will always be present in your intestines, it's when there's an overgrowth of either one of them that it can impact health.

For example, candida alone can produce 70+ toxins as waste, which harm your mitochondria, liver, kidneys, brain, and immune system.

Intestinal bacterial overgrowth can do the same.

The other issue is that when the "good bacteria" gets crowded out by some of the "bad bacteria," like clostridium difficile, your immune system begins to suffer.

You may also begin to develop symptoms of bloating, gas, constipation, diarrhea, IBS, heartburn, GERD, acid reflux, acne, headaches, anxiety, mood disorders, auto immune issues, and fatigue.

And these are just the tip of the iceberg, since 80% of your immune system resides in your gut, then the ramifications of an imbalanced gut spread through the entire body.

Another gut bug that's often overlooked (sometimes for fear of finding one) is parasites. Parasites are so much easier to get than we think…

And parasites aren't only a concern for those traveling to an area of the world with improper water decontamination. You can catch a parasite from undercooked meats and fish, or even just at your local salad bar. It's estimated that 25% of the population (1 out of every 4 people) is walking around with a parasite without even knowing it.[49]

I've worked with many people who have had tapeworms, giardia, ova, cysts, and other parasites in their intestinal tract that were making them sick and they didn't even know it. It was only after I had them begin my parasite cleansing protocol that they expelled the parasites and could begin the healing process.

As I said before, if you're truly looking for the hidden underlying root causes for why you can't get well, lose the weight, or fix your digestion, you must look deeper into healing the gut.

ARE WE BEING SLOWLY POISONED?

After reading that Top 10 Toxins list there are many people that believe we are intentionally being systematically poisoned by pharmaceutical companies (BigPharma), corporations (BigCorporate), and food manufacturers (BigFood).

I personally do not hold that view.

Don't get me wrong. I do know they are aware of the harm they are causing and we are without a doubt being slowly poisoned… But I believe it's more a side effect of greed and not malice.

I personally believe that most companies put profits above people.

What they care about, ultimately, is making more money and to do that, it's easier to create synthetic man-made chemicals that can be patented and cheaply manufactured. This cuts product costs and allows them to increase their profit or undercut the competition – or both.

The problem is that this outlook is short-sighted.

So short sighted that it's typically too late before these companies are told that their new "wonder drug" or product actually causes harmful side effects.

This is often why you won't find the heads of these companies using their own products. It's the same reason why former presidential administrations won't speak out about the harmful effects of pesticides and GMO foods, but they choose to feed themselves and their family organic.

It's this veil of secrecy or non-transparency that is the most damaging.

Another example is the dental industry's stance on "silver" amalgams containing mercury and aluminum, which are known to be harmful—toxic and poisonous in fact, to human health.

Although they've always agreed that you need dispose of these fillings as a hazardous toxic material, they somehow felt it was safe to put in people's mouths in the first place, right?

Now they're in too deep and can't say it's harmful for fear of the repercussions of lawsuits and general distrust of conventional medicine—all the fall-out created by telling the truth.

This same point holds true with the military using DDT during the Vietnam war to knock the leaves off trees. The side effect was that it is a synthetic neurotoxin that never biodegrades. This means this chemical will be around forever in our soil, water, and air slowly destroying our nervous systems.

Which is why we have to do our own homework. A lot of the truths we need to be maximally healthy can never be told because of legal ramifications and the loss of the almighty profit.

OUR NEW REALITY

If this is our new reality—if this *must be our reality*—well then, we must find a means of protecting ourselves.

This is my firm belief.

I am someone who believes very much in choosing to be optimistic and that optimism is very good for mental and physical well-being.

But I also live with both feet firmly planted on the ground. And today, more than optimism, we need to be forewarned and forearmed to protect ourselves and our families from the dangers lurking all about us.

The great news is there *is a solution*.

It's a solution that works, and it's been proven to effectively reduce our chances of developing any number of diseases, as well as improving our mood and transforming our body into the healthy lean machine it's supposed to be!

The following chapters are dedicated to helping you finally get well, lose weight, and feel alive again – but, before we uncover the exact protocol I use in my practice, I need you to understand how and why some people get sick, why some get cancer, or become overweight while others seem to remain just fine.

It is in this next chapter that I will explain the revolutionary discovery called, "*The Rain Barrel Effect.*"

Once you understand this innate biological feature in all of us, it will become clear why we can go from fit, happy, and healthy to sick, tired, and overweight…

Part 2
The Rain Barrel Effect

The Real Reason We Become Sick, Tired, & Overweight

> *"Americans of all ages are carrying around over 219 toxic chemicals in their body at any given time…"*
>
> - Center for Disease Control, 2009 *Fourth National Report on Human Exposure to Chemicals*

TOTAL TOXIC LOAD

The first time I heard the term "total toxic load," also referred to as "total body burden," I was intrigued, but didn't fully understand what it meant.

I wanted to research more to find out how such a thing could exist and how it might be impacting our health. What I found is that just from normal metabolic cellular processes, we humans are constantly building up waste in our body.

Just like the smoke that comes from burning wood in a fire, every single time we eat or produce energy, our cells and digestive system create waste by-products. And it's like this for every system in our body.

But all that waste must be properly eliminated to stay healthy. So, our body must tend to that waste. That's a primary duty of the body.

But what I don't think I grasped fully for some time, because of the sheer magnitude – and the frightening implications for our health – is what happens when our body not only has to deal with the natural waste we create, but it now has tens of thousands of toxic chemicals that it must find a way to expel without doing harm to the internal system (liver, kidneys) that filters all this waste.

All these invisible and insidious toxins that hide in our atmosphere become more for our body to filter.

Quite simply, this is the point: Our bodies are not designed, or properly equipped, to filter out paint fumes, synthetic fragrances, plastics, and other man-made chemicals.

How much can any one organ filter before harm begins to occur within that organ?

What our liver does, for example, in the phase I pathway, is try to take a toxin and turn it into a non-toxin by using another compound or mineral in the body to reform it in a way. But when it cannot find a way to turn that toxin into something that appears "waste friendly" through this kind of transformation into something more like an excess vitamin or mineral, it passes it off to the phase II pathway.

In a sense, it says, "I cannot handle this one, can you?"

When the phase II pathway cannot process the toxin then it stores it somewhere, like adipose (fat) tissue.

As a result, our body continues to accumulate these particles and store them away in hopes of preventing harm to the internal organs, like the liver and kidneys, that have to attempt to transform toxins into non-toxic substances before they can excrete them – a process that is highly exhaustive to these organs as well.

The problem is we eventually meet our upper limit. Each person's limit, or threshold, is dictated by their age, genetics, gut microbiome, lifestyle, food intake, and all the other factors that will be explained in the coming DESTRESS Protocol™.

NATIONAL GEOGRAPHIC ARTICLE

Many people still refute that toxins are an issue. The reason is that most of the toxins, although very real, are nanoparticles that can't be seen.

Scientists know these nanoparticles exist, but only the larger ones, like gold nanoparticles, can actually be observed.

And of course, we can't see the processes happening inside of our bodies. But, even for the greatest skeptic, the existence and damaging effects of these poisons in the body are irrefutable for anyone that would like to do a lab test for themselves.

One of the most well-known examples of this occurred when a self-proclaimed skeptical journalist, David Duncan (pictured below), from *National Geographic Magazine* decided to see what was really going on with our internal toxicity levels.

The article was originally published in October, 2006, and was titled, *"The Pollution Within: How Modern Chemistry Keeps Insects from Ravaging Our Crops, Lifts Stains from Carpets, and Saves Lives. But the Ubiquity of Chemicals is Taking a Toll."*

The article talks about how toxicity in the environment is now inescapable and how

> "Each year the U.S. Environmental Protection Agency (EPA) reviews an average of 1,700 new compounds that industry is seeking to introduce.
>
> Yet the 1976 Toxic Substances Control Act requires that they be tested for any ill effects before approval only if evidence of potential

harm exists – which is seldom the case for new chemicals. The agency approves about 90 percent of the new compounds without restrictions. Only a quarter of the 82,000 chemicals in use in the U.S. have ever been tested for toxicity."

(Note: This was written in 2006 and the number of chemicals has greatly increased.)

The *National Geographic* writer then went on to perform the ultimate test to see if he was harboring any of these toxic chemicals in his body.

After all, he felt like he was a healthy individual. Why would he have any dangerous toxins or metals in his body? There couldn't really be any really dangerous chemical accumulation that could cause disease or cancer down the road, could there?

For the purposes of this article he was tested at the world renowned, Mount Sinai Hospital in New York City, by Dr. Leo Trasande.

A SKEPTIC'S RESULTS

Here are the results of the dozens of toxins found in his body as quoted by Duncan:

> "Some of them date back to my time in the womb, when my mother downloaded part of her own chemical burden through the placenta and the umbilical cord. More came after I was born, in her breast milk. Once weaned, I began collecting my own chemicals as I grew up in northeastern Kansas, a few miles outside Kansas City.
>
> My test results read like a chemical diary from 40 years ago. My blood contains traces of several chemicals now banned or restricted, including DDT (in the form of DDE, one of its breakdown

products) and other pesticides such as the termite-killers chlordane and heptachlor. The levels are about what you would expect decades after exposure, says Rozman, the toxicologist at the University of Kansas Medical Center.

My childhood playing in the dump, drinking the water, and breathing the polluted air could also explain some of the lead and dioxins in my blood, he says. [Later in life,] I encounter a newer generation of industrial chemicals—compounds that are not banned, and, like flame retardants, are increasing year by year in the environment and in my body.

Sipping water after a workout, I could be exposing myself to Bisphenol A, an ingredient in rigid plastics from water bottles to safety goggles. Bisphenol A causes reproductive system abnormalities in animals. My levels were so low they were undetectable—a rare moment of relief in my toxic odyssey.

And that faint lavender scent as I shampoo my hair? Credit it to phthalates, molecules that dissolve fragrances, thicken lotions, and add flexibility to PVC, vinyl, and some intravenous tubes in hospitals. The dashboards of most cars are loaded with phthalates, and so is some plastic food wrap. Heat and wear can release phthalate molecules, and humans swallow them or absorb them through the skin." [2]

David Duncan, like all others who decide to put their skepticism to the test, ultimately came to realize that total body burden is a real thing and that it is the invisible factor that we need to correct in order to get healthy.

I could also go on and on about how David is not just a one-off case study, but instead, I'm going to share with you how you too can run a simple at home test in order to discover your own toxicity levels.

But first, I want to provide you with one more form of scientifically tested evidence that should end the toxic accumulation debate once and for all…

THE 10 AMERICANS STUDY

When I was first learning about toxicity it made me upset and angry to think that corporations were knowingly putting harmful additives into our foods and dumping chemicals into the environment.

But this next issue really pushed me over the edge and I got mad enough and started writing this book, compiling study after study. I wanted to do something to inform as many people as I could and help prevent a lifetime of being chained to diagnoses and pharmaceutical drugs.

We don't have to live our lives fat, tired, and doomed for dis-ease.

Here's where the science gets shocking:

Right now, every newborn baby that comes into this world is already filled with man-made toxins that weren't even a part of our world just 150 years ago. It is these same chemicals that can cause birth defects, autism (now 1 in 68), cancer, and other diseases.[1] It's unspeakable to think that we know these toxins cause these childhood issues, yet nothing is being done.

A video and study called *"10 Americans"* by the Environmental Working Group (EWG) was released showing that before a child is even born they already have approximately 287 toxins in their blood and tissues. This data came from 10 newborns whose parents gave permission to have their toxin screens done at birth.[1]

(The 10 Americans video and EWG study above can be seen in its entirety at StephenCabral.com/10-americans)

An average of 200 chemicals was found in each newborn. 47 of those toxins were consumer ingredients such as cosmetics. 212 were from industrial chemicals and pesticide breakdown products. (Keep in mind only about 400 total chemicals were actually being tested for in this study. Thousands of others may have been found if larger parameters were used.)

Many of the toxins that were found in these newborns included plastics, flame retardants, and other chemicals that disturb the brain function, IQ, nervous system, and hormones of the baby. Some of these chemicals like DDT, believe it or not, have actually been banned for over 3 decades, but are still being found in blood and urine samples. The reason for this is that certain chemicals never fully degrade in the environment.

So, as we've now discovered, it's not a question of whether you have disease creating toxins inside your body, but rather which ones and how much.

That's why I encourage everyone to find out exactly how bad his or her toxic burden is.

HOW TOXIC ARE YOU?

Lab testing is a very powerful tool that most Functional Medicine practitioners use in active clinical practice.

It allows both the patient or wellness client to see for themselves what the underlying root cause is for why they're suffering from any number of health issues. There is literally a lab for each specific issue and I will provide those in the appendix and RBE resource page.

One of the best ways to begin to take control of your health is to have your toxicity levels tested by a Functional Medicine practitioner. You can purchase the lab from your doctor or on your own right online.

Here's a sample lab of what those results may look like:

Toxic Compounds

Metabolite	Result µg/g creatinine	Percentile

Herbicide

16) 2,4-Dichlorophenoxyacetic Acid (2,4-D)	3.8	LLOQ 0.20 — 75th 0.50 — 95th 1.9

2,4-Dichlorophenoxyacetic Acid (2,4-D) is a very common herbicide that was a part of Agent Orange, which was used by the U.S. in the Vietnam War. It is most commonly used in agriculture on genetically modified foods, and as a weed killer for lawns. Exposure to 2, 4-D via skin or oral ingestion is associated with neuritis, weakness, nausea, abdominal pain, headache, dizziness, peripheral neuropathy, stupor, seizures, brain damage, and impaired reflexes. 2, 4-D is a known endocrine disruptor, and can block hormone distribution and cause glandular breakdown.

Pyrethroid Insecticide

17) 3-Phenoxybenzoic Acid (3PBA)	4.3	LLOQ 0.30 — 75th 1.0 — 95th 5.8

Parent: Pyrethroids - Including Permethrin, Cypermethrin, Cyhalothrins, Fenpropathrin, Deltamethrin, Trihalomethrin
Pyrethrins are widely used as insecticides. Exposure during pregnancy doubles the likelihood of autism. Pyrethrins may affect neurological development, disrupt hormones, induce cancer, and suppress the immune system.

Metabolite	Result Creat mmol/mol	Percentile

Marker for Mitochondria Function

18) Tiglylglycine (TG)	0.75	LLOQ 0.04 — 75th 4.7 — 95th 11

(This is just page 1 of the over 100+ toxins tested for using a simple at home urine test.)

When you run this toxicity lab called the GPL-TOX, by Great Plains Laboratory, the higher your levels represented by the black bar, the more toxins you've been exposed to and you're holding onto, which are continuing to build up in your system. Over time, these chemicals can cause (or have already caused) major health issues.

DO YOU SUFFER FROM?

This particular lab company especially recommends running this test if you suffer from any of these conditions linked to total toxic load:

- Alzheimer's Disease
- Amyotrophic Lacteroclerosis (ALS)
- Anorexia Nervosa
- Anxiety Disorder

- Apraxia
- Arthritis
- Asthma
- Attention deficit (ADD)
- Attention deficit with hyperactivity (ADHD)
- Autism
- Autoimmune disorders
- Bipolar disorder
- Cancer
- Cerebral palsy
- Chronic fatigue syndrome
- Crohn's disease
- Depression
- Developmental disorder
- Down Syndrome
- Epilepsy
- Failure to thrive
- Fibromyalgia
- Genetic diseases
- Irritable bowel syndrome
- Learning disability
- Mitochondria disorder
- Multiple sclerosis
- Obsessive compulsive disorder (OCD)
- Occupational exposures
- Parkinson's disease
- Peripheral neuropathy
- Schizophrenia
- Seizure disorders
- Systemic lupus erythematosus
- Nervous tic disorders
- Tourette's syndrome
- Ulcerative colitis

BRINGING LAB TESTING TO THE MASSES

I remember, the first time I ran this lab. I was shocked to find that I had a few elevated levels of toxic chemicals.

After all, I eat healthy, take my nutritional supplements, exercise, etc. However, I tested high on exhaust fume particles. Considering I live in downtown Boston and walk everywhere, it shouldn't have been a surprise. Every day I'm exposed to car, bus, and train exhaust that lingers in the air which I, of course, breathe in.

So, although I'm now clear of all the others after detoxing my body, I understand that if I'm going to live and work in the city, I must continue to keep my system as clean as possible. This is why I continue to follow my own DESTRESS Protocol ™ to stay well.

The 2nd lab test you may decide to run is a Hair Tissue Mineral Analysis. It looks at toxic heavy metals such as mercury, lead, aluminum, and arsenic. I've also found it quite useful in testing high copper levels in cases of ADD, ADHD, Autism, skin issues, fatigue, and other mood and learning based health issues.

Again, you can ask your Functional Medicine Practitioner to run this lab for you. Or, you can purchase them online and run them yourself. The choice is always yours to do what you feel is right for your body at this moment in time.

Although the lab test David Duncan ran cost about $15,000 over a decade ago, I'm happy to say you can now run the same lab for just a few hundred dollars. You also don't need to go to a fancy hospital, or even get your PCP to approve it. You can run this simple urine and/or hair based lab right at home and then mail in your sample to the lab. Just a few weeks later you will get your results, as well as a plan of action to improve your health.

If lab testing is too expensive right now, at the end of this chapter I'll also be providing you with a Toxicity Quiz to find out just how toxic you are from a symptomatic standpoint. I believe in both symptoms based questionnaires, as well as state-of-the-art lab testing. If possible, you may want to do both.

Now that hopefully you agree that most every person on this planet is likely infected with dozens of toxic chemicals, I'd like to explain exactly how that leads to the outward symptoms of disease, weight gain, and an overall wearing down of your body and mind. It is only after understanding this concept that you can then reverse the dis-ease process.

THE RAIN BARREL EFFECT EXPLAINED

When I was 20 years old sitting in the waiting room of my allergist's office and suffering miserably from red, swollen shut, dry itchy eyes, post nasal drip, and chest congestion, I picked up an article lying amongst the magazines.

I had already been dealing with allergies most of my life and had read quite a bit on how to "deal" with them. However, this article immediately caught my attention. I didn't know it at the time, but it would trigger a new mindset that would be the beginning of my healing journey.

This article mentioned a phrase in passing that I had never once heard uttered by doctors, specialists, or anyone inside the medical community. To this day, it's still rarely uttered…

It's called the *"Rain Barrel Effect."*

What it is, and how it eloquently explains how we get sick, age, gain weight and lose our vitality is life changing. Once you know the how and why you got where you are right now, you can then finally begin to heal.

The *Rain Barrel Effect* is the answer you've been looking for. It explains the "mystery illnesses" like the one I had where your blood work looks fine, but you're still sick and tired. It also answers the question of why you may have that auto-immune, skin, join pain, headache, or other officially diagnosed disease.

This is one of the biggest concepts in natural health and medicine that's very rarely, if ever, talked about…

The best way to think about how and why you got sick, overweight, or just feeling like "blah," is to picture a rain barrel, or just a bucket.

A rain barrel is used to catch water from gutter runoff and hold onto it every time it rains. No one ever notices the rain is filling up the barrel until, of course, the barrel overflows…

It's at that point that the barrel needs to be emptied or it will no longer function properly. Instead of the barrel serving a healthy purpose, it will instead spill over onto your garden or patio and create unwanted issues such as a dead spot of grass in your backyard.

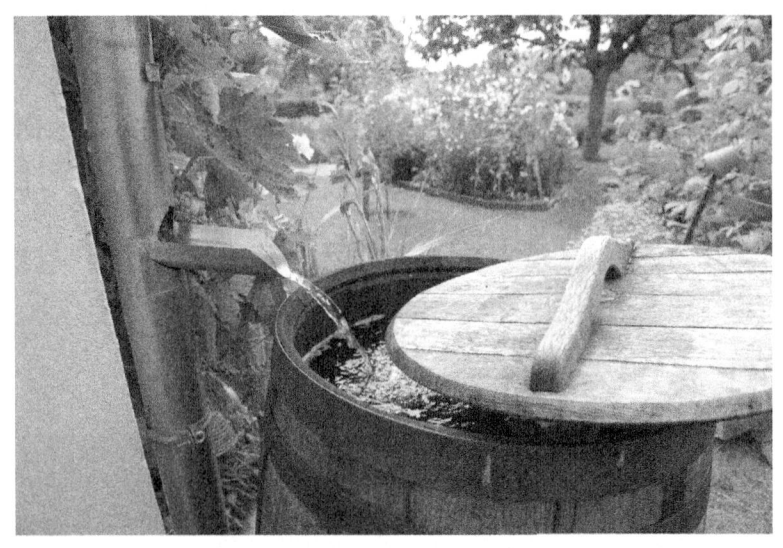

(Image of a rain barrel filling up with water from gutter runoff.)

The same theory holds true for our own bodies. Over time, we accumulate toxins. Some, as mentioned earlier, come from the environment and are man-made. Others come from candida, bacteria, parasites, stress hormones, or other internal metabolic processes.

What happens is that when these natural and synthetic toxins float around in our blood they must be disposed of. This then takes energy, the proper nutrients, rest, and a well-functioning liver to filter out the harmful substrates. As long as your body is getting everything it needs then the process continues to run smoothly and maintain equilibrium.

The problem is that as the years pass, we accumulate more and more toxins and our bodies begin to run low on certain reserves. Our bodies then begin to lose the internal battle and our rain barrel begins to fill up faster. But even as your rain barrel is filling up you still may not see any initial symptoms of not feeling well.

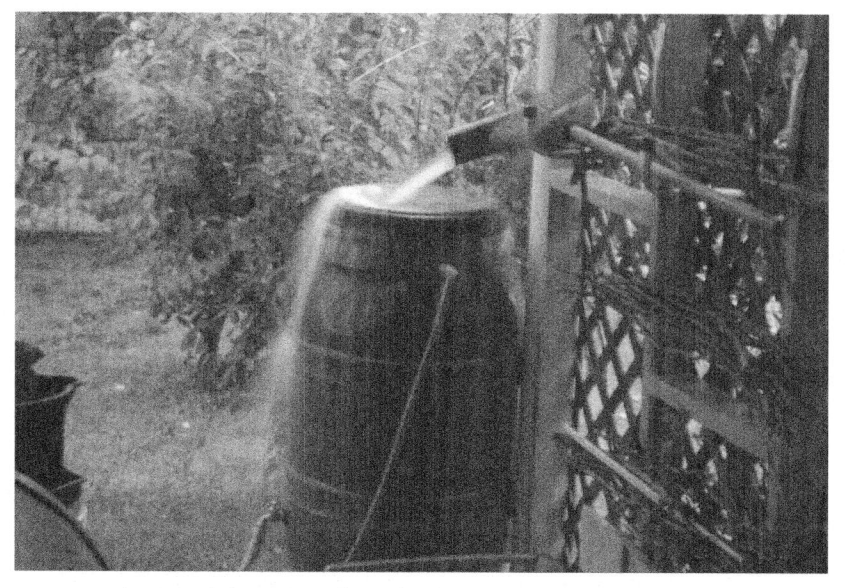

(Image of a rain barrel overflowing when it's met its capacity.)

Most often, noticeable external symptoms do not arise until your rain barrel begins to overflow. Unfortunately, just like a real barrel that catches the rain you won't know it's full (unless you lab test) until it's spilling over the sides. The reason for this is at this point your body, and the barrel, can no longer keep up with the demands placed on it. It has no more reserves left.

It's also at this time, that you will begin to feel the outward symptoms of your internal systemic imbalances. You may see or feel pain, skin issues, headaches, fatigue, inflammation, weight gain, a loss in vitality or really any sign of poor health.

You may even be diagnosed with a disease or specific health condition such as high blood pressure, high cholesterol, auto-immune, chronic fatigue, fibromyalgia, allergies, asthma, Alzheimer's, Parkinson's, or any other set of symptoms we give a name to for insurance and drug prescription purposes.

YOU ARE NOT YOUR DISEASE

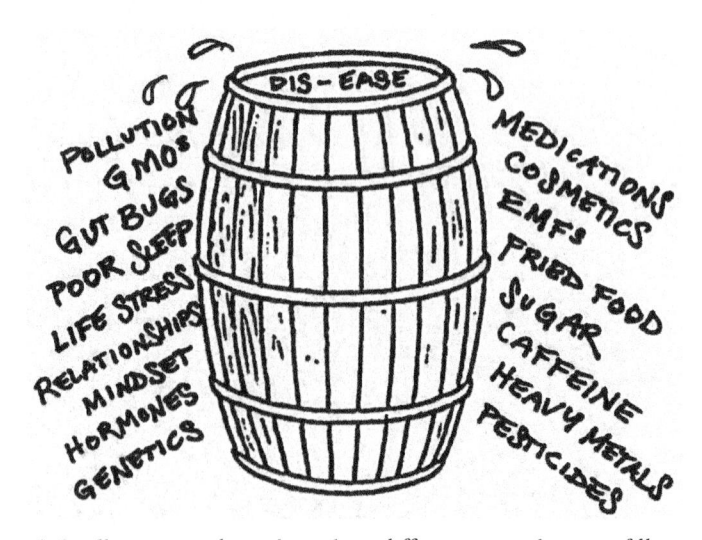

(The illustration above shows how different toxins begin to fill up your rain barrel, which when overflowed results in symptoms we call a disease – Then we then medicate those symptoms.)

A rain barrel will of course continue to take on more water, but not without spilling additional contents. It will continue like this until the owner empties its current load. It has no other choice and neither does your body. Luckily, just like the rain barrel, you too can empty your barrel and lighten your toxic load!

As I said, when I first learned about this discovery I knew it was going to be an important part of me figuring out how to recover from my own "mystery illnesses" that the best doctors and specialists in the world couldn't figure out. Little did I know, over a decade later it wouldn't just play a role in me getting well, it turned out to be the answer that I and many others were searching for...

CHRONIC DISEASE EXPLAINED

No chronic disease, illness, cancer, or any other health issue happens overnight. It is a slow gradual wearing down of our body's defenses that eventually gives way to poor health.

Even conventional medicine has now come around to this thought process, and in 2013 the *National Institute for Health* published an article by Andrew W. Campbell on *Autoimmunity and the Gut*, which detailed the pathology of the dis-ease. The problem is that we usually only see the outcome of the dis-ease – But not the rain barrel filling up. We notice the symptoms. And those symptoms such as fatigue, weight gain, join pain, skin issues, infertility, auto-immune, digestive, cancer, etc. are the end results.

The image depicted below is something we commonly use in Functional Medicine to show patients how they get sick. It also explains to them how they are not their disease. Their disease is merely their body's expression of an inward imbalance – or overload of toxins that it is trying desperately to fight and eliminate, so it can maintain homeostasis within the body.

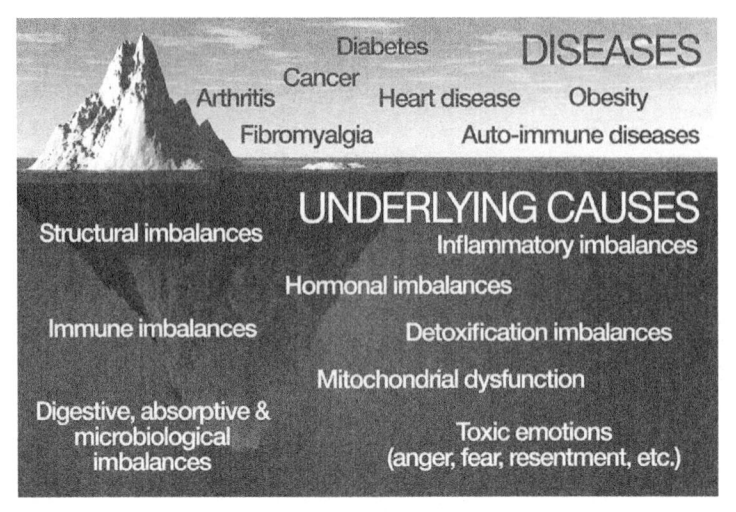

DISEASES
Diabetes, Cancer, Arthritis, Heart disease, Obesity, Fibromyalgia, Auto-immune diseases

UNDERLYING CAUSES
Structural imbalances
Inflammatory imbalances
Hormonal imbalances
Immune imbalances
Detoxification imbalances
Mitochondrial dysfunction
Digestive, absorptive & microbiological imbalances
Toxic emotions (anger, fear, resentment, etc.)

(The symptoms that we see are only the tip of the iceberg.)

Each person will always have their own genetic predisposition to what they may be susceptible to for health issues if their total toxic load becomes too great. For example, in my family most everyone gets rheumatoid arthritis and digestive issues. However, no one seems to get Hashimoto's, lupus, multiple sclerosis or other auto-immune issues.

The interesting concept, though, is that these dis-ease names are all different expressions from the same malfunctions in the body. We see them as different diseases, but they are not. They are simply different manifestations of an imbalanced body trying desperately to rebalance itself. This is why the symptoms you're dealing with are not the disease itself. Most of the time, symptoms are the outward sign of your body trying to "right the ship" and heal itself.

For example, most people believe when they get a fever they have to reduce it at the first sign. However, the fever is not the sickness. The fever is your body trying to speed up the flow of white blood cells and raise your body temperature in order to naturally kill viruses or an infection. It is only when a fever becomes too high that we should try to lower it.

Your body knows what it is doing and wants to help you heal. This is why suppressing symptoms will never lead to healing. It can't. The reason is that when you treat the symptoms you are missing the target completely, since the symptoms are a response of the body to an underlying root cause issue.

THE RAIN BARREL EFFECT CONNECTION

The *Rain Barrel Effect* (RBE) has not only had a powerful impact in my own life, but I've now used it many years later to help thousands of people I care for in my practice…

I am able to help them see how over a period of years the stress of school or work, raising a family, accumulating toxins, taking prescription drugs, and not eating well has begun to take its toll. They begin for the first time to see that their dis-ease did not just happen overnight. It was a slow wearing down of their body's ability to maintain equilibrium when faced with an accumulation of toxins as described in Part 1.

The more interesting realization is that with many conditions such as an auto-immune disease, psoriasis, alopecia, and others there is often a triggering event.

I've discovered through thousands of office appointments this triggering event is usually something very personal. It means a lot to them (or it did at the time) and it's often still difficult to talk about. I've also seen it mainly be tied to a relationship difficulty, break up, divorce, loss of a loved one, or some other major stressful time in their life. It can be work related, but usually the work must mean a great deal to them.

The best way to think of this situation is that the person's rain barrel had already been filling up and then they were exposed to a massive "storm." It was this stressful storm that then wiped out their reserves and filled up their rain barrel the rest of the way.

THE 3 TRIGGERS FOR DISEASE

After completing over 250,000 appointments in my wellness, weight loss, and anti-aging practice I've come to see that all dis-ease states in the body have 3 main cascading events

Once these 3 triggers for disease have taken place in the body you will then see and feel the outward symptoms of the inner turmoil. This is what the Rain Barrel Effect looks like in the real world.

THE 1ST TRIGGER: GENETICS

Right now, many MDs or specialists will tell you that your cholesterol, auto-immune, blood pressure, etc. is just "genetic" and there's nothing you can do about it except medicate…

That couldn't be further from the truth. However, before I explain that let's talk about how and why your genetics do matter.

Inside your DNA lies building blocks called single nucleotide polymorphisms (SNPs). Inside of your genome you have about 10 million of these SNPs (pronounced "snips"). It is these SNPs that predict how your body will react to medications, drugs, alcohol, stress, weight gain, toxins, and what your susceptibility is to various diseases.

For example, in my family we have a very difficult time regulating inflammation. We are also prone to higher levels of adrenal stress hormone output. And when it gets too high it can also cause a dis-ease state. In my particular family, this equates to the auto-immune disease rheumatoid arthritis, allergies, Th1/Th2 immune imbalance, and gut dysfunction like SIBO.

And although the mechanisms are the same, you may have inherited a different genetic code leaving you susceptible to Hashimoto's, lupus, psoriasis, alopecia, or any number of other diseases. It is our DNA that allows for the expression of these diseases if our rain barrel overflows...

An old saying in Functional Medicine goes like this, "Genetics loads the gun, but it's the environment that pulls the trigger." Our next trigger explains what that really means.

THE 2ND TRIGGER: ENVIRONMENT

Your environment is the 2nd trigger to becoming unwell, run down, or gaining weight. The interesting thing is that your environment is composed of more than you think. It's not just the pesticides, GMO foods, heavy metals, and polluted water. It's also what's happening inside your body.

That's the environment that we don't always pay attention to since it's hidden away inside of us. This means that the stress hormones, neurotransmitters, cellular waste, and other metabolic toxins from our internal workings build up. Additionally, one of the most predominate triggers for disease is increased intestinal permeability (leaky gut).

The reason why I've mentioned this multiple times now is that it has literally been implicated in over 90% of all disease. That's because when you have leaky gut, the foods you eat, as well as bacteria and yeast can move directly into your blood stream. This then turns on an exaggerated immune response and causes massive imbalances and inflammation within the body.

Unless you've run an Organic Acids Test or another lab to look for candida or bacterial overgrowth you may be missing the most important factor in finding a major root cause to your current state. *(I will provide recommendations and write ups on all the labs in the resource section in the back of this book.)*

So even though we've now set the stage for dis-ease in the body (either mental or physical) we still need one more trigger to fill up your rain barrel enough for the disease state to take place…

THE 3RD TRIGGER: THE "EVENT"

There's always a reason why…

I've had the amazing fortune to be able to work with thousands of people in my Functional Medicine practice. In almost every single case I've been able to tease out what their triggering event was before they finally saw the overflowing of symptoms in their life.

Remember, your genetics simply sets the stage, but it's the environment that allows for the expression of those genes. The last step is the proverbial "straw that broke the camel's back." This is where you've left yourself open to this devastating dis-ease state.

This is also why you'll often see yourself go from nagging digestive issues, headaches, occasional inflammation, joint pain, constipation, a few skin rashes, or other initial symptoms, to a major eruption of a sick state.

In my practice this is what I see most often as the triggering events:

- Massive stressful event (break up, death in family, etc.)
- Heavy metal exposure (dental work, vaccine, polluted water, etc.)
- Virus or Infection (Epstein Barr, Herpes, etc.)
- Pesticide (recently sprayed golf course, backyard, etc.)
- Food poisoning (foreign bacteria exposure)

DON'T WAIT FOR YOUR RAIN BARREL TO OVERFLOW

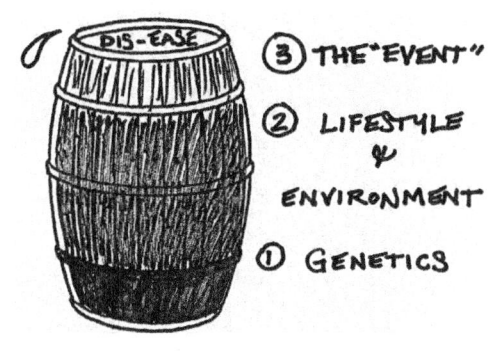

(It is this last triggering event that overflows your rain barrel where your symptoms now spill over and we feel "sick.")

(Note: For a more in depth look at these 3 triggers for disease please see the link for my podcast episode #410, the Cabral Concept, which goes in depth on this issue: StephenCabral.com/410)

Next up, I want to share with you what these 3 triggers look like in the real world and how they work against you unless you are aware of their influence.

MY RBE STORY

Everyone has their own RBE story and although we experience it in our own unique way, the undertones are always the same.

In my own life, at 17 years old, I had already been filling up my own rain barrel. It was my 3rd year of taking antibiotics on a daily basis for minor acne that many teenage boys experience. However, my dermatologist prescribed amoxicillin twice a day indefinitely. Each month I filled my prescription not knowing that it was wiping out my gut bacteria and along with it, my immune system.

At this same time, I was taking my SATs for college, choosing an out-of-state school, preparing to uproot from my good friends, relationships, family, and everything I knew in life. This in itself was a major stressor, and when you add on top of it more stress from sports competitions, working out, dating, my after-school job, and homework, you can see how my rain barrel would be getting full…

Now add to those high levels of stress lots of poor eating and a lack of sleep and you can begin to realize how I was ripe for some triggering event to cause my rain barrel to overflow. (Remember, even though I was pushing my body to the limit, I still had no outward symptoms – I felt great!)

I should also add that my diet consisted of mainly cereal for breakfast, sandwiches with bread and processed deli meat and cheese at lunch, and pasta or meat for dinner. After dinner, I was also allowed to have a bowl of my favorite neon-green mint chocolate ice cream. For beverages, I'd drink juice with breakfast, Kool-Aid during the day, and a tall glass of cold milk with each meal. This was far from a picture of healthy eating!

Although no one knew it at the time, I clearly had a gluten and dairy food sensitivity issue, which was resulting in frequent sinus infections, ear infections, mucous production, and allergies.

Most cold New England Winter's would be spent with me catching a cold, getting a sinus infection with post-nasal drip and then taking another course of a different antibiotic. To me though, all of this was a "normal" part of being a kid, since no one had ever taught my parents or myself otherwise…

Then one day I contracted Epstein Barr Virus. Of course, I left myself wide open to this virus since my imbalanced immune system was suffering from the massive leaky gut consequences induced by the over 3,000 capsules of amoxicillin (as well as acid-blockers) I had already swallowed by 17 years old and from the high amounts of stress, exercise, over-work, poor eating, and lack of sleep.

That was my triggering event and when I woke up that November morning, my life would change forever. Since my immune system had been totally wiped out in some areas (I had a SIgA white blood cell count of 0 and overactive in others, my body couldn't regulate itself.

This then led to greater health issues such as auto-immune joint pain, fibromyalgia, debilitating brain fog, chronic fatigue, and Addison's Disease.

MY RAIN BARREL - CAUSE & EFFECT

I've never shared this story before since it was such a dark time in my life. And the truth is that I spent over 5 years searching for an answer that conventional medicine couldn't give me. I was angry, frustrated, anxious and depressed thinking about the fact that I may have to live this way for the rest of my life.

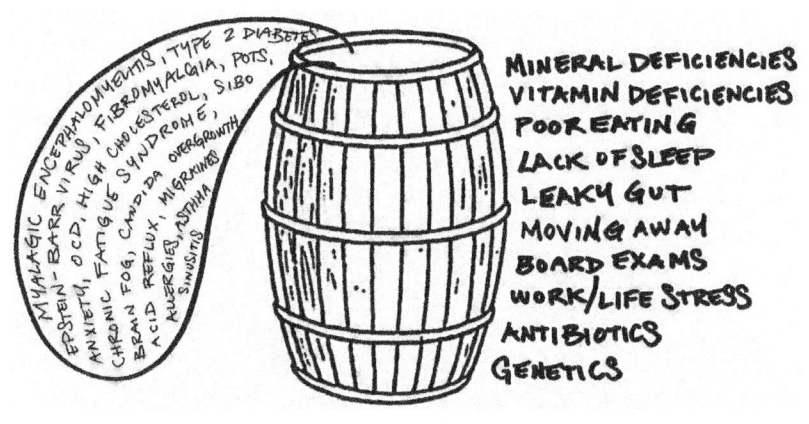

(This illustration depicts my personal rain barrel filling up with "toxins"(right side) and then overflowing with a dozen diagnosis's (left side) of dis-ease states.)

The good news is that I eventually had a chance encounter with an alternative medicine doctor that opened my eyes to a whole new world of healing.

That's how I began my own recovery and what ultimately led me on the path to now.

I will share more about my mentor in the next section and you will receive the plan you need to begin your own wellness, weight loss, or anti-aging when I explain my DESTRESS Protocol™. But now, I'd like to clear up some misconceptions related to improper dis-ease diagnosis.

INFLAMMATION IS NOT A ROOT CAUSE

Many health enthusiasts and practitioners alike that are doing good work are mistakenly treating inflammation as something to remove from the body.

Inflammation is never a root cause issue. It is a symptom that is caused when your rain barrel gets too full. Inflammation is a sign of an underlying health condition that has given way to an immune response or tissue damage (often both). This means that by trying to suppress the inflammation you are not working on the true underlying root cause. And without rebalancing the underlying issue, you will always be treating inflammation.

This is why I don't like to use a lot of natural anti-inflammatories in my practice. I like to gauge our progress based on physical symptoms as well as lab results. Therefore, if I'm suppressing symptoms by using prolonged curcuminoids (turmeric) or another natural supplement, I am masking tell-tale signs of disease and health.

Now of course I don't want anyone to suffer, so in the short-term I have no issue with using some natural anti-inflammatories to relieve pain. However, I want to make sure that in the long-term we all realize inflammation is a helpful sign showing us how well our bodies are doing internally.

Now that we know inflammation is not a foe, let's look at how particular diseases "grow" in the body…

A SUMMARY OF CHRONIC DISEASE STEMMING FROM THE RAIN BARREL EFFECT

Now that you know why you or a loved one has gotten to this point in your life, let's talk a little more about how your specific health condition may have come about.

We all deal with sickness, diseases, and our health in different ways. Sometimes our symptoms seem unique to us, but I'd like to share an example below giving a brief overview of how particular dis-ease states arise.

I hope that you can then begin to make correlations to your own health or weight issues and see that no matter what you suffer from, it too has an underlying root cause connected to your rain barrel being too full and your body being imbalanced.

THE AUTO-IMMUNE CONNECTION

As I mentioned in passing earlier, all auto-immune conditions are just different manifestation of our genetic predispositions when the environment has become right for them to be expressed.

Right now, 90% of all auto-immune conditions have their root cause stemming from gut based dysfunction. This means that either heavy metal, bacterial, parasite, or candida infestations have caused an imbalance in the gut bacteria. That gut dysbiosis (more bad than good bacteria) compounded with increased gut wall permeability (leaky gut) causes an exaggerated immune response.

This immune response causes an imbalance in Th1 vs. Th2 immunity (amongst others such as Th17), which allows for a heightened inflammatory reaction. For example, in rheumatoid arthritis (RA), a strong predisposition by your body to create CD4 and CD8 immune cells lends itself to a larger degree of tissue destruction. This is mainly explained as a function of a "confused" immune system, or something called, "molecular" mimicry which asks the immune system to attack our own cells and tissues because they look like that of a toxin that has been marked as an antigen ("invader").

However, one major fact is being overlooked – Right now in medical science we are developing stronger microscopes, which are enabling us to look deeper inside the cells. In the case of people with auto-immune issues like RA, scientists are finding something they've termed "micro-bacteria" or "nano-bacteria."

This is bacteria that is so small, it's gone undiscovered until now. But, discovering these bacteria inside the cell may now explain why our immune system is actually attacking those cells that are harboring foreign toxic bacteria that have come from the gut, foods, the environment, or other pathogens.

In auto-immune diseases, an imbalance is further provoked by heavy metal and other toxic accumulation such as mercury and fluoride. It is metals and toxins like these that can then go on to cause Hashimoto's or thyroid dysfunction. In this case, it is due to the fact that vital nutrients such as iodine and selenium are needed for proper thyroid function and those minerals may get blocked. (This was further explained in Part 1, but you can find out more about the 4 toxins [mercury, arsenic, aluminum, bromines] that affect the thyroid at StephenCabral.com/593)

All of these underlying imbalances in the body that cause poor health reinforces the idea that to reverse an auto-immune condition or other diseases, we must first make the body a hospitable place to live. This means clearing out as many heavy metals, synthetic man-made environmental toxins, gut pathogens, pesticides, and other chemicals keeping us sick.

Luckily all of this is possible and you will soon discover for yourself how to remove the obstacles that are hidden inside of you and keep you from enjoying the healthy happy life you deserve!

GUT ISSUES

Nearly 2/3rds of my Functional Medicine practice is caring for people with gut issues that have never been helped by conventional medicine. They have been diagnosed with terms like IBS, IBD, Crohn's, Colitis, SIBO, diverticulitis, etc.

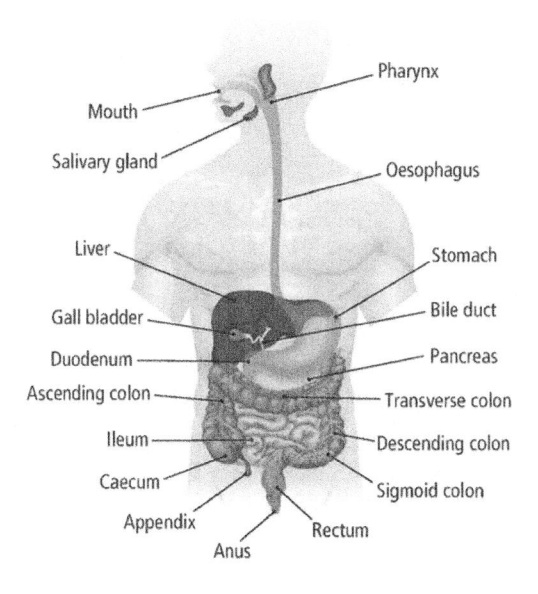

(In order to properly heal all dis-eases and weight issues you must ensure that the bacteria in your gut microbiome is balanced and that you've removed the yeast and bacterial overgrowth.)

The problem is that all of the diseases above are really just names for a set of symptoms. And those symptoms are simply different ways of saying that you have "irritable bowels." Did you really go to your doctor, and GI specialists, to have them tell you that you have irritable bowels? I'm pretty sure you already knew that…

The unfortunate part is that conventional medicine is only trained to give you more antibiotics or anti-spasmodic drugs for many of the issues above.

Antibiotics only compound the dis-ease, further irritate the bowel, and aggravate symptoms because previously prescribed antibiotics for various illnesses are often times cause of your current gut issues in the first place!

The reason is, of course, that when you take antibiotics, they don't just kill the "bad" bacteria, but they also wipe out a lot of the "good" bacteria as well.

This is an major issue since when you wipe out the natural bacteria in your gut, you are creating imbalances in your gut microbiome. Plus, the good gut bacteria are used to help absorb food, manufacture vitamins, and ensure harmful chemicals don't make their way into your blood stream. Without a positive balance of healthy gut bacteria to pathogenic bacteria and yeast strains, you will feel all of the symptoms of intestinal discomfort.

The way to heal the gut is to understand how the *Rain Barrel Effect* caused you to suffer from these issues in the first place. After working with thousands of people with every gut issue imaginable, I'd like to share with you a straight forward example of the how they got into this position in the first place.

THE BEGINNING OF GUT IMBALANCES

Please keep in mind that the reason why I am so focused on the gut is that, as stated before, it comprises 80% of your immune system.

During a vaginal birth a mother passes on her bacteria to her child. If the birth was by c-section or the mother's microbiome wasn't as healthy as it could be, children may start life off with an imbalanced gut. This often sets the stage for a less than perfect immune system, which in conventional medicine warrants a course of antibiotics every time the child gets a cold or infection. These antibiotics further weaken the gut and in time, this can lead to additional food sensitivities.

These sensitivities cause inflammation from offending foods, which further exacerbate intestinal lumen openings, also known as leaky gut. And, because of the antibiotic use, candida and other pathogenic yeast strains tend to overgrow, while more negative forms of bacteria like e. coli are permitted to proliferate as well.

With your microbiome out of balance, the intestines stop properly breaking down and absorbing food particles as well, which leads to a general weakening of the body due to poor nutrient absorption (even if you're eating a healthy diet). Plus, when your intestinal ecosystem is imbalanced your ability to produce happy, calming neurotransmitters like serotonin becomes compromised leaving you feeling tense, anxious, overwhelmed and irritable.

None of this happens overnight. Many people make it well into adulthood before they begin to see the outward symptoms of the inward imbalances caused by the cumulative weakening of their gut as a whole.

This is why by the time people see me in my practice their first complaint isn't just aggravated bowels. They are in pain, frustrated, unhappy, and at a loss for how to end this vicious cycle. Many think probiotics are the answer, but unfortunately most people are not informed on how and when to properly use probiotics.

Adding more probiotics (bacteria) to a gut with already too much yeast or bacteria in it will only exacerbate gut issues and is not recommended until you remove the yeast and bacterial overgrowth first – because adding more toxins or toxic bacteria to an already full rain barrel is not always the answer.

The DESTRESS Protocol™ will teach you how to *"Empty Your Rain Barrel™"* before adding more of the good, healthy bacteria back in.

TOXIC FAT

In my practice, I work with a lot of women and men trying to lose weight and keep it off permanently. The problem is that we've been brainwashed by the media to approach this issue in a totally unproductive manner. They've become obsessed with all the wrong issues, like reducing calories, going sugar-free, or eating no carbs or high fat.

But let's think about why obesity rates continue to rise despite a constant bombardment of trendy new diet plans, food options and many of us becoming much more conscious of what we eat. Long-term weight loss and maintenance seems to be a bit of an enigma in our society and I believe after reading this you will never look at weight loss as simply a "calories in, calories out" problem ever again…

As we've reviewed previously when your liver and body cannot keep up with the plastics, pesticides, heavy metals, and other chemicals in your blood it will look to push them through your skin or store them some place. One of the places our body prefers to store harmful chemicals is our fat cells.

These fat cells make up what is referred to as adipose tissue. Our fat is essentially a convenient compartmentalized storage unit. Our blood shuttles these toxins to our fat stores. and then locks the door, sealing the toxins in that fat tissue. Although this shields us from the toxins, in a sense, and keeps us temporarily safe from immediate harm, there are repercussions. We get fat. Literally, our adipose tissue begins to swell.

So, one of those side effects of your internal toxicity is weight gain. As the toxins build up in your fat stores, the adipose tissue grows – this is an actual increase in body fat even though some of it is fluid. You start to feel puffier, more swollen and your body looks softer—like you're losing muscle tone.

I speak about this topic all the time on my podcast and I let people know that often weight gain is not a consequence of eating too much or exercising too little.

The weight gain issues we're dealing with in our present day has mostly to do with toxic foods, hormonal metabolic imbalances, and the environment we live in, which subsequently causes inflammation and chemical storage in fat cells. This then leads to unnecessary water weight gain as a result. Practitioners and patients alike often confuse this *toxic water weight* with actual fat weight.

But these are two very different problems—detoxifying versus weight loss – and without the detox, the weight will stay on the body. So these two issues must be treated individually in order to achieve long-term weight management success.

TOXIC WATER WEIGHT

One of the other issues with toxic water weight gain from chemicals and hormones is the stubbornness of trying to take it off.

If it were really just about *calories in, calories out,* you could just eat less and exercise more and the weight would simply melt from the body. However, as many know and have struggled with it, it's just not that simple.

Some people eat far less than their friends, but they still can't lose the weight. There is, of course, a reason for this, and a large part of it has to do with this viscous cycle of toxicity.

As endotoxins build up from imbalanced gut bacteria, hormonal metabolite byproducts, and/or being exposed to outside exotoxins like heavy metals and plastics, your inflammation and cortisol levels rise and all these toxins will deposit in you fat cells.

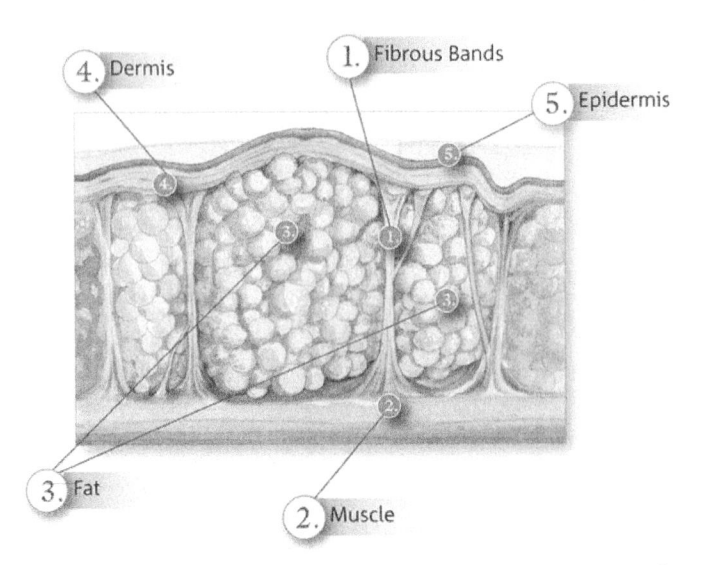

1. Fibrous Bands
4. Dermis
5. Epidermis
3. Fat
2. Muscle

(Cellulite is a perfect example of toxins accumulating in your fat cells and causing uneven swelling in your connective tissue.)

As fat cells expand and grow, estrogen levels typically rise as well. This leads to additional weight gain and water retention which, in turn, makes it more difficult to lose weight and decrease inflammation. It's a self-perpetuating cycle that must be broken.

When viewing weight gain from a *Rain Barrel Effect* perspective, we can easily see that an increase in fat tissue on the body is due to an overflowing of your rain barrel.

This could be from too many calories from toxic processed food, but most likely, it's your environment and internal exposure to toxins like stress, imbalanced gut bacteria, hormonal imbalance and dysregulation, lack of sleep, pesticides, plastics, and other toxin accumulation.

The end result is an accumulation of adipose (fat) tissue stores.

The problem is that most people and books are only telling you to lower your carbohydrate intake or manipulate your diet or to simply exercise more – as if these steps alone will undo all the damage your body undergoes daily just from living in a toxic world. Perhaps steps like these were great cure-alls before the industrial revolution. But not now.

This view completely disregards your external and internal environment, which is why most people aren't getting the results they want. Until you start to *Empty Your Rain Barrel*^{TM}, you will always struggle with keeping the weight off. The good news is you now know how you got here and what can be done to heal the very root cause of all your problems.

(For additional *Rain Barrel Effect* examples on almost every dis-ease such as high cholesterol, high blood pressure, acne, psoriasis, eczema, headaches, migraines, fatigue, high/low thyroid, anxiety, depression, estrogen dominance, cancer, PTSD, Alzheimer's, Parkinson's infertility, ADD/ADHD, and many more please visit StephenCabral.com)

RELAPSING

The Rain Barrel Effect also explains how and why people relapse even after getting well and losing the weight.

I spent close to a half a decade going back and forth between getting well for a few weeks to a few months and then relapsing only to feeling sick, tired, depressed, and broken down again. I had no idea what was working to get me well or what was causing the relapse back into illness. What I didn't know back then was that the *Rain Barrel Effect* held the answers to all these questions.

Now I know that the reason I relapsed so often was that even when I was feeling well, I had only emptied my rain barrel just enough to get rid of my symptoms. Therefore, I was always on the edge of overflowing my barrel again… All it would take was one night of missed sleep, a stressful exam, a night out with friends, or a food I was sensitive to and I'd be right back where I started!

This is why merely removing the symptoms with pharmaceutical drugs, anti-inflammatory herbs, or other supplements is never the long-term solution.

Plus, although I tell my private clients that they will most likely be feeling alive and well again within just 21 days (due to t he emptying of their rain barrel), the deeper healing takes place after about 12 weeks, as your cells begin to turn over, and your body begins to renew itself from the inside out.

This is the innate beauty and amazing healing power of your body. You simply need to give it a helping hand. First, help it to remove the toxins and then provide it with the nutrients it's missing in order to regenerate. This is truly the answer you've been searching for!

HOW TO BEGIN HEALING

In this next chapter, I will begin to explain how to get well, lose the weight, and finally feel alive again!

This journey took me close to 20 years of study, a doctoral degree in naturopathy, and reading thousands more books but even with all that I still didn't fully have the answer…

It was only when I spent my first naturopathic internship overseas on a small island Southeast of India did I discover the answer – But before we get to "my search for answers," I want to make sure you find out your own *Rain Barrel Toxicity Score* by taking this short quiz on the next page.

How full is your rain barrel?

Let's find out!

The RBE Toxicity Quiz

How Full Is Your Rain Barrel?

> *"In industrialized societies cancer is second only to cardiovascular disease as a cause of death. But in ancient times, it was extremely rare There is nothing in the natural environment that can cause cancer."*
>
> - Professor Rosalie David

Most people that live with aches, pains, fatigue, and health issues think this is just a normal part of aging…

But nothing about living that way is normal and it's unfortunate we've been led to associate the aging process automatically as a forgone conclusion that our body is going to start to break down and we're going to have to suffer from disease, weight gain, flabby muscles, and fatigue.

It truly doesn't have to be that way and it's my life's work to show you how to reverse your current state, but before we get there I'd like you to assess where you're presently at.

To do that, I've given you my private Functional Medicine Detox Assessment to find your level of total toxic load and build up.

HOW TO TAKE THE QUIZ

To complete the toxicity questionnaire and find your personal results score, simply fill in the blank ___ with a 0, 1, 2, or 3 depending on your typical symptoms

0 = Never feel this symptom
1 = Feel this symptom 1-2 times per month
2 = Feel this symptom weekly
3 = Feel this symptom daily

HEAD

___ Headaches/Migraines
___ Dizziness/Faintness
___ Neck tension
___ Cloudy head

SINUS

___ Nasal congestion (stuffy nose)
___ Allergies (seasonal or daily)
___ Mucus
___ Sneezing
___ Nose blowing

EYES

___ Dark circles under eyes
___ Bags under eyes
___ Itchy eyes
___ Discharge or watery eyes
___ Blurred vision
___ Crusted eyes upon waking

EARS

___ Itchy ears
___ Discharge or drainage from ears

___ Ringing in ears, tinnitus
___ Excessive wax build up
___ Blocked or muffled hearing

TEETH

___ Pain in gums or teeth
___ Bleeding gums
___ Silver fillings (Score with a 3 if you have any metal fillings)
___ Metal crowns or Root canals (Score a 3 for crowns or root canals)

MOUTH

___ Canker sores
___ Cold sores (herpes virus)
___ Cracking on lips
___ Discolored lips
___ White film on lips upon waking or after eating

TONGUE

___ Red dots on tongue
___ Sides of tongue have dents ("scalloping")
___ White, yellow, or brown coating on tongue
___ Cracks or lines on tongue

GLANDS

___ Swollen lymph nodes (neck, armpits, or groin)
___ Difficulty swallowing
___ Loss of voice
___ Swollen ankles or wrists/hands/fingers

BREATHING

___ Chest tension
___ Inability to get enough air in
___ Chest congestion
___ Chronic cough
___ Clear throat a lot
___ Voice hoarseness

WEIGHT

___ Difficulty losing weight
___ Gain weight easily
___ Feel swollen or puffy
___ Retain water
___ Binge or compulsive eating

JOINTS/MUSCLES

___ Pain in joints
___ Muscle stiffness
___ Limited range of motion
___ Muscle weakness/Loss of strength
___ Arthritis

SKIN

___ Acne
___ Hair loss
___ Flushing/Hot flashes
___ Dry, flaky skin
___ Excessive sweating

___ Hives or itchiness
___ Psoriasis, eczema, ringworm or skin rashes

SLEEP

___ Inability to fall asleep
___ Can't stay asleep/Wake up frequently
___ Nightmares
___ Heart racing at night
___ Night sweats

ENERGY

___ Tired upon waking
___ Daytime or afternoon fatigue
___ General lack of energy
___ Apathy
___ Lack of ambition or drive
___ Hyperactivity (can't sit still – always doing something)
___ Restlessness (feel uncomfortable with quiet)
___ Tap feet or shake leg or hands when seated
___ Decreased libido or sexual function

DIGESTION

___ Get tired after meals (especially lunch)
___ Bloating
___ Gas
___ Belching/Burping
___ Heartburn or indigestion
___ Diarrhea
___ Constipation

___ Stomach or intestinal pain
___ Nausea or vomiting
___ Stomach sticks out more as day progresses

MIND

___ Lack of concentration
___ Easily distracted or lose train of thought
___ Difficulty making decisions
___ Brain fog
___ Stuttering or difficulty putting together sentences
___ Uncoordinated or drop things
___ ADD/ADHD or learning disabilities

EMOTIONS

___ Anxiety
___ Overwhelm
___ Irritability
___ Anger or rage
___ Dark thoughts
___ Sad for no reason
___ Mood swings
___ Depressed
___ High-strung
___ Seasonal Affective Disorder (SAD)

IMMUNITY

(Score each question below with 10 points if you answered yes)
___ Frequent colds (Do you get more than 3 illnesses a year?)
___ Allergies (Do you have environmental or food sensitivities?)
___ Pneumonia *(Have you had pneumonia in the last year?)*

___ Diagnosed disease *(Do you have a diagnosed disease?)*
___ Unexplained illness *(Do you have an unexplained illness?)*

TOTAL SCORE

___ Grand Total Score (add up your total points from above)

SCORING RECOMMENDATIONS

Take a look at your overall quiz results and see which health sections you seem to be doing the best and what areas need some work. The higher score areas are where you have underlying imbalances that must be corrected.

After adding up your total point score see what toxicity stage you're at below:

STAGE 1: 0-9 POINTS

Congratulations it looks like you're doing great! You appear to be well and it seems like you have your health under control. Just make sure you are not filling up your rain barrel with continued stress, lack of sleep, poor eating, etc.

My recommendation in terms of detoxification at this point is only a seasonal 7-day detox to keep up with and remove the continual accumulation of environmental toxins. Do also try to incorporate a healthy daily routine as shared later in this book in order to stay well and balanced.

STAGE 2: 10-19 POINTS

It looks like you're doing pretty well overall, but you're starting to see the effects of hidden toxicities expressing themselves on the outside as symptoms. It's also at this point that you may be moving towards a dis-ease state unless you begin to Empty Your Rain Barrel™.

A formal 7, 14, or 21-day detox is advised and then seasonal detoxes after that to maintain optimal health and balance. I also highly recommend incorporating the daily healthy living routines shared later in the DESTRESS Protocol™.

STAGE 3: 20+ POINTS

Your body is now showing signs of toxic overload and total body burden. Most likely, you are feeling the effects of this toxicity in your daily life in terms of inflammation, lowered vitality, lowered mood, and less overall "get up and go."

A 21-day detox is recommended followed by seasonal 7, 14, or 21-day detoxes to decrease toxic accumulation until you reach a score of 10 points or less. At that point you can simply drop down to one 7-day detox seasonally/quarterly. This is also the time to pay special attention to each step in the DESTRESS Protocol™ coming up soon.

HOW TO DO A FUNCTIONAL MEDICINE DETOX

How to complete a 7, 14, or 21-day Functional Medicine detox will be explained in the upcoming chapters and summed up in the last section of the *Rain Barrel Effect* for easy reference. You will also learn the daily detox methods you can use to lighten your total body burden, as well as alternative non-toxic recommendations to keep yourself healthy going forward.

Lastly, each time you complete a 7, 14, or 21-day detox please retake this RBE Toxicity Quiz to see how your score has decreased. And remember, my personal total toxicity score on this test used to be well over 100 pts! Now, it remains below 10 points and I want to show you how to do the same.

(Note: On the online resource page for this book, I will attach a PDF download of this same quiz in order for you to print out copies whenever you'd like.)

IT'S TIME TO DISCOVER THE 6,000 YEAR OLD SECRET

Up next, I reveal the *6,000 year old secret,* which ultimately led to me creating my DESTRESS Protocol™.

To be honest, I had studied Ayurvedic Medicine for many years, but had no idea about the power of these rejuvenation treatment protocols before I landed on the tiny island of Sri Lanka.

This next part of my journey will always bring back special memories from when I finally discovered the truth about how to get well, lose weight, and feel alive again -

Now it's time to share that with you!

Part 3
The Search for Answers

A Skeptic's Journey

"Because we cannot scrub our inner body we need to learn a few skills to help cleanse our tissues, organs, and mind. This is the art of Ayurveda."

- SEBASTIAN POLE

By the time I was in my mid 20's, I had gotten used to being given half-answers.

After all, my amazing and caring parents took me to all the best medical specialists, but I was never given an actual explanation for what was wrong with me. I was 5 years into my healing journey, still with no end in sight. I felt defeated, completely frustrated, and skeptical.

I believed this idea of the *Rain Barrel Effect* could hold the answer to what I and millions of others were suffering from, but I still didn't know what to do about it. All I kept going back to was the thought that if a rain barrel could fill up, there had to be a way to empty it - right?

The issue is that modern, conventional medicine doesn't work this way. They're good at adding more to the body in terms of drugs and therapies, but removing toxins doesn't seem to even be an area of interest.

This left me with no choice but to seek out alternative medicine options.

After reading a particularly interesting book, *My Doctor Says I'm Fine, So Why Do I Feel So Bad?*, I decided to contact the author. It's not a very well-known book, but it spoke to me.

To be honest, I don't even know how I stumbled upon this book, yet little did I know, it was to be one of the greatest discoveries of my life...

The author, Margaret Smith Peet, is a Naturopath and Ayurvedic practitioner. She studied directly under Vasant Lad, who was the foremost authority on Ayurvedic Medicine in the United States. Dr. Peet actually transcribed his lectures into the two textbooks used in his classes. She also studied Functional Medicine and blended this with her traditional Naturopathy background.

On a whim, I contacted Dr. Peet by email. I was desperate and somehow, I believed in her words. What she said in that book resonated with me deeply. I also believed her unique background would be able to provide some answers to my ongoing issues.

She agreed to do a consultation with me in Camden, Maine, so I took the 3-hour bus ride up there one Friday morning. It was to be a meeting I would never forget.

I had never met anyone like her before in my life. She somehow knew exactly what I was going through, why I was going through it, and how I got there in the first place.

She introduced me to Traditional Naturopathy, Functional Medicine, Orthomolecular Medicine, and Genomics all in one day!

MY MENTOR'S ADVICE

After multiple meetings with her over that winter and as my health began to improve under her guidance, she decided to turn the tables. She said she had saw something in me from the first day we'd met.

She told me I too would make a great Naturopathic Doctor and that I should think about going back to school that coming Fall. I still don't know the reason to this day, but her words had such impact on me that I still get misty-eyed when I recount the story…

Maybe it was because of her belief in me when I felt very alone, or maybe it was because deep down, I knew my life's work would be dedicated to relieving the struggles of those like me who were suffering illnesses that conventional medicine offered no clear answers – Those living without hope like I once was.

I will never forget Dr. Margaret Smith Peet and I hope that my work today is making her proud. It was, indeed, her guidance and teachings that finally got me here.

Once I applied all I had learned from Dr. Peet to my own life, I never looked back. I threw myself completely into studying naturopathic medicine with fervor and dedication.

I was so determined to succeed, to help others as I was helped, that I decided to intern overseas to learn everything I could from every successful practitioner of naturopathic medicine in every country and culture that I could. I wanted to learn more about Chinese Medicine, Ayruvedic Medicine, all of it. I wanted to see what ancient medicines still had to teach us and how modern practitioners of cultures with rich histories of natural cures now viewed curing modern maladies by combining ancient wisdom with new advancements in science.

At this point, I had read over 3,000 books written by brilliant American authors on all things health, wellness, anti-aging and psychology and now it was time to see what the rest of the world was doing

I figured that since conventional medicine in the US didn't hold all the answers we were searching for, it was time to see what other places could teach us. This instinct couldn't have been more right. On my very first internship overseas, I was in for the biggest awakening of my life...

THE AWAKENING

When I arrived on the tiny island of Sri Lanka, I didn't know what to expect. I had heard so much of the Ayurvedic clinic there that serviced over 200 patients and wellness guests at a time. During my time there, I was to learn from the top doctors and work with individual patients on their ailments from a modern-day Ayurvedic perspective.

I had already read well over 100 books on Ayurveda and been mentored by one of the best Ayurvedic teachers, but nothing prepared me for actually putting this ancient science into practice.

I was now in the real world seeing the effectiveness of these treatments on some of the sickest people I'd ever encountered.

Secretly, this was exactly why I was here though...

The constant skeptic in me wanted to see which form of medicine actually helped people get well. Would it be Ayurvedic Medicine, Traditional Chinese Medicine, Traditional Naturopathy, OrthoMolecular, or Functional Medicine?

What I saw there in Sri Lanka were people who came in with debilitating diseases like rheumatoid arthritis and were moving pain free within 6 weeks.

I saw others with full body psoriasis come in with open sores and leave with fresh, clear skin. Hundreds of other cases of every dis-ease you could think of were going into "remission." I was seeing with my own eyes what I had only read about in books.

However, from a conventional medicine perspective none of these healing cases should have been possible. We shouldn't have been able to get patients these types of results without the newest drugs from the best labs of conventional medicine. But we did.

And it was on an island in the middle of nowhere off the Eastern tip of India cut off from most of the world.

The fact that I was seeing these results caused me quite a bit of confusion and mental agony. I just couldn't wrap my head around why no one else knew about these ancient secrets that had been working for over 6,000 years! How could people be getting well and the word hadn't spread like wildfire? These, and hundreds of other questions just like them, kept me up at night.

I knew I had witnessed something that I couldn't just bury in the back of my mind and forget about. It was then that I made a promise to continue my studies overseas and keep seeking out the best of all forms of medicine and then unite them into one practice. It was a tall order, but I knew this is what Dr. Peet believed I would one day do.

MY SEARCH WAS OVER

After 2,400 clinical internship hours in Sri Lanka, India, China, Europe, and the US, studying every form of traditional and state-of-the-art medicine you could think of, it was now time to put all I had learned into practice.

The challenge was, how do I blend close to a dozen forms of medicine into one clinical setting?

For this answer, I had to distill the very best from every discipline and then unite it into one practice. I also had to come up with a system that worked consistently every time.

I went back the beginning and I asked myself what was the basic foundation that every non-conventional form of medicine used to get people well again?

The answer was and has always been to return the body to a state of equilibrium. This means cleaning out all the pathogens, bacteria, yeast, viruses, chemicals, excess hormones, and toxins that shouldn't be there.

It was only at this point that the body could then take on more.

It makes perfect sense in hindsight, right?

To fill up a cup that is already full, you must first empty some of its contents.

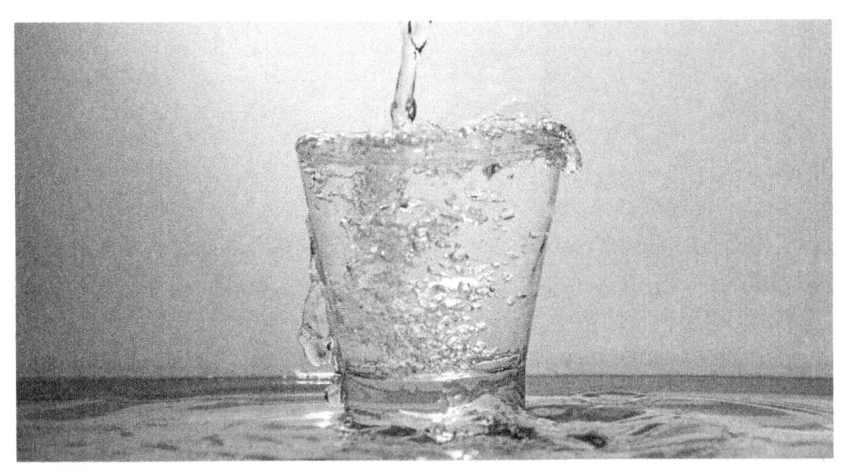

(Sometimes the best form of medicine is subtractive – not additive.)

It was at this time that I came up with the concept that you must *Empty Your Rain* Barrel™ to get well, lose the weight, or live longer!

I finally understood we were all speaking the same language no matter what the form of natural medicine being practiced. There were just different metaphors and ancient disciplines going about it in slightly different way – but all saying the same thing.

In order for the body to get well, lose weight, and feel great, you must remove the blockages keeping you from getting there.

It's the only way.

Somehow, Ayurvedic Medicine knew this over 6,000 years ago…

THE 6,000-YEAR-OLD ANSWER

When people ask me how the people I saw in those Ayurvedic clinics got well so quickly, I share with them one defining truth of ancient and natural medicine.

I call it a secret because even though it is available to anyone that wants to use it, it's locked away in Ayurvedic texts, which are not very approachable from a Western perspective. By this I mean the wording and methodologies are foreign to us.

We have been brought up in a Western perspective and because of that our minds have been molded to think in one specific pattern. This is why I had such a hard time intellectually "buying in" to the treatments.

Sure, I had read about them in books, but it wasn't until I saw the healing with my own eyes that I verified the results and became a believer. So what is *the secret*?

PANCHA KARMA

It's called Pancha Karma (PK). It literally means 5 actions.

The process of Pancha Karma seeks to detox, cleanse, and rejuvenate the body, mind, and consciousness.

It is meant to help:

- Eliminate toxins
- Balance the body

- Strengthen the immune system
- Reverse the effects of stress
- Enhance vitality and energy
- Improve metal clarity
- Deepen relaxation & well-being
- Renew & rejuvenate the entire body

Although 6,000 years of continued use as the oldest form of medicine in the world should be enough, luckily for science-based skeptics like myself, there is literally a pile of research showing Pancha Karma does exactly what it states.

(Note: To read more about Ayurvedic scientific research please see the 656 page researched textbook called, *Scientific Basis for Ayurvedic Therapies*, as well as *Ayurvedic Healing: Contemporary Maharishi Ayurveda Medicine and Science. Second Edition.*)

The 5 treatments for Pancha Karma are all different, but all aimed at doing one thing. It's all centered around detoxification. Therefore, special types of diet, lymphatic massage, sauna/steam, enemas, and oil treatments are given to the patient. The traditional purifying treatments include:

ABYANGA

Before beginning any of the 5 specific treatments in Pancha Karma, the cornerstone of this rejuvenation and body-balancing therapy is a form of massage called, Abyanga.

Although there are multiple variations of therapeutic massage in Ayurvedic Medicine, Abyanga is the most revered. It is a gentle rhythmic massage done by 1 or 2 therapists. And the uncanny thing about this type of massage is that it is *the original form* of manual lymph drainage. I was literally shocked (after studying the Vodder Method of lymphatic massage) that this style of massage was not created in the 1930s, but rather 6,000 years ago in India.

Regardless of who takes credit for it, Abyanga or manual lymphatic drainage has a tremendous effect on your health.

ABYANGA MASSAGE BENEFITS

- Nourishes the entire body—decreases the effects of aging
- Imparts muscle tone and vigor to the dhatus (tissues) of the body
- Imparts a firmness to the limbs
- Lubricates the joints
- Increases circulation
- Stimulates the internal organs of the body
- Assists in elimination of impurities from the body
- Moves the lymph, aiding in detoxification
- Increases stamina
- Calms the nerves
- Deepens sleep
- Enhances vision
- Makes hair (scalp) grow luxuriantly, thick, soft and glossy
- Softens and smoothens skin; wrinkles are reduced
- Pacifies Vata (anxiety) and Pitta (aggression) and stimulates Kapha (stagnation)[1]

A Pancha Karma treatment massage, or self-massage (taught in later in this book) is often completed daily in the clinic. This helps to speed up the detoxification process, as well as enhance the effects of the additional PK treatments listed below:

DIET

During a detox like Pancha Karma, typically a vegetarian or vegan diet is prescribed to cut down on the amount of new toxins coming in from animal tissue meat. Also, by not eating meat, patients do not need to divert as much energy for digestion and therefore, healing can take place faster. Mainly fruits, vegetables, and dishes like Kitchari (mung beans/lentils and rice with ghee) are eaten. Specific herbs are also used for detoxification support.

VAMANA

This treatment helps to eliminate, Kapha (phlegm) and Pitta (heat) symptoms, or mucous build up in the body. It is highly effective for bronchial asthma, allergic bronchitis, rhinitis, sinusitis, migraine, hyperacidity, indigestion, anorexia, obesity, overweight, dyslipidemia, diabetes mellitus, acne vulgaris, psoriasis, eczema, urticaria etc.

Although not used in the United States, it is a process of bringing mucous into the stomach by drinking milk followed by emesis therapy. This means patients actually vomits in a controlled environment to remove the mucous from the upper respiratory area. I know it's hard to believe in our Western culture, but the results have been studied and proven to be effective from a modern-day medical perspective.[2]

VIRECHANA

The Sanskrit word, Virechana, translates to purgation. This is when a patient is given specific foods and herbs to help loosen bile and detox the liver emptying into the colon where a bowel movement is then induced. Inducing multiple bowel movements, usually in the form of loose stool, typically happens after a few days of preparation

BASTI

Besides Vamana, Basti was the least favorite (but often the most effective) treatment in the Ayurvedic clinics I interned and studied at. A basti is a "medicated" enema. This means an herbal water or oil based decoction was inserted into the rectum of a patient. Sometimes, the patient would be instructed not to expel the herbal liquid and allow it to absorb into the body, but mostly the enema would induce a bowel movement within about 15-minutes. With the bowel movement would come released intestinal toxins.

NASYA

This treatment involves applying an Ayurvedic herbal oil in the nose along with a special facial massage to open up the sinuses. Typically, after the oil is placed in the nasal cavity, a steam inhalation is given. It's remarkably effective for upper respiratory issues and easy to replicate at home.

(Note: While on one of my trips to India I was suffering from an upper respiratory illness as well as allergies and Nasya treatments were incredibly effective at reducing my pain, swelling, and symptoms.)

ADDITIONAL TREATMENTS

There are many other Ayurvedic treatments such as Shirodhara (warm oil applied to forehead) for calming the mind and Svedana treatments like steam and sauna, which are used for sweating out toxins. Both of these (and others) are used as part of all Pancha Karma treatments to purify the body by eliminating toxicities through the skin, bile, bowels, urine, upper respiratory tract, and the lungs.[3]

A Pancha Karma study at the Institute of Science, Technology and Public Policy at Maharishi University of Management in Fairfield, Iowa in collaboration with a special laboratory at Colorado University revealed:

1. PCB and DDE levels appear to be unexpectedly high in the general population, and may actually be increasing. This is surprising since these toxicants were banned decades ago in many countries.

However they have not disappeared from the environment since they have half-lives that last several years. Also they are still entering the food chain through imports.
2. Within days Pancha Karma treatment eliminated a large proportion of these fat-soluble toxins from the body. Without this intervention, the expected drop would be only a fraction of 1%.
3. This study shows banned PCBs and agrochemicals in blood were reduced 50% by Ayurvedic detoxification procedures.[4]

A DEEPER UNDERSTANDING OF PANCHA KARMA

I believe my job is to be an educator first and a natural health doctor second. This means I seek out the best research and treatments available, no matter how complex (as is Ayurvedic Pancha Karma) and then make it actionable for the real world.

So when I was studying Ayurvedic Medicine overseas, I asked the doctors running the clinics a lot of questions. We would sit for hours and I would share what I had studied in the US and they would then relate it to Ayurvedic Medicine. Again, it was eye opening how what we consider new, state-of-the-art testing, diagnosis, and treatments were already understood 6,000 years ago. This means we're literally rediscovering old information today…

However, I still wanted to know what Ayurvedic Medicine held as its fundamental healing process. I was told multiple times that it all centered around purifying the body through detoxification. Ayurveda believes that disease comes from an accumulation of "ama" (toxins).

Therefore, every Ayurvedic method used was chosen in order to purify and detox the body. However, I later discovered special emphasis was placed on "cleaning the blood." This turns out to be a key component that cannot be missed…

THE MISSING COMPONENT

There are thousands of "detoxes" being sold on the market, but most miss the crucial concept of how to effectively detox. In Ayurveda, as well as modern day science, we know the fastest and best way to detox is by supporting the liver, which is the main organ that cleanses your blood.

This was the secret to many of the Ayurvedic treatments. They detoxed the liver with certain herbs and amino acids, which support what's called Phase 1 and Phase 2 liver detoxification. This is such an important and critical role in getting you well that I'd like to explain it to you in more detail.

Every 6-minutes all the blood in your body is circulated through your liver. It is literally the filter for your blood. Just like a home or car air filter, your liver removes the impurities out of its environment so that you're not exposed to their harmful properties. The issue is, of course, that filters become dirty, congested, and clogged.

Your car, vacuum, or home air filter gets cleaned or switched out every few months with continued use, but for some reason we've forgotten to maintain our own body's filter. This point alone literally holds the key to getting back your health since adding more and more to your body will not matter until you can get your liver functioning properly again. If anything, adding more (even when using healthy products) may actually make you worse due to your total toxic load and the inability for your liver to keep up.

The good news is that we know without a doubt how best to support the strongest detoxifying organ of the body. By using a detoxifying diet and adding in specific nutritional supplements to support the liver we can help it function faster and more efficiently.

LIVER DETOXIFICATION

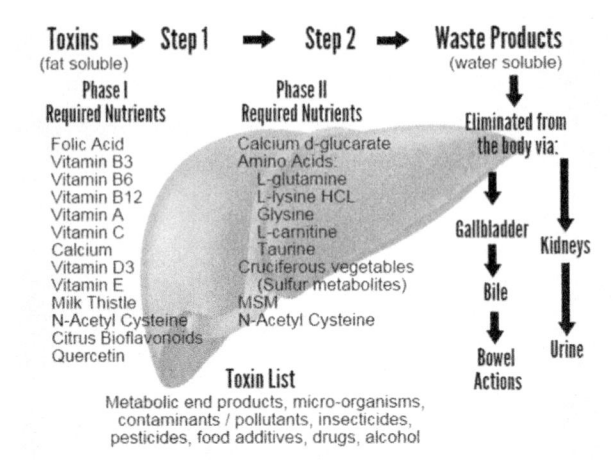

Toxins (fat soluble) → **Step 1** → **Step 2** → **Waste Products** (water soluble)

Phase I Required Nutrients
- Folic Acid
- Vitamin B3
- Vitamin B6
- Vitamin B12
- Vitamin A
- Vitamin C
- Calcium
- Vitamin D3
- Vitamin E
- Milk Thistle
- N-Acetyl Cysteine
- Citrus Bioflavonoids
- Quercetin

Phase II Required Nutrients
- Calcium d-glucarate
- Amino Acids:
  - L-glutamine
  - L-lysine HCL
  - Glysine
  - L-carnitine
  - Taurine
- Cruciferous vegetables (Sulfur metabolites)
- MSM
- N-Acetyl Cysteine

Eliminated from the body via:
Gallbladder → Bile → Bowel Actions
Kidneys → Urine

Toxin List
Metabolic end products, micro-organisms, contaminants / pollutants, insecticides, pesticides, food additives, drugs, alcohol

(Notice all the vitamins, mineral, antioxidants and amino acids above needed to keep your liver functioning optimally.)

As you can see from the image above your liver is always detoxing and cleaning your blood every second of the day. However, it may not be operating at top performance if it's missing or low on any of the nutrients essential for proper function. This is why Functional Medicine detoxes work so well. They supply you with the must-have nutrients vital for your liver to do its job.

PHASE 1 DETOX

It's important to distinguish between the two phases of liver detoxification. During phase 1 of liver detox your liver is taking fat soluble metabolites (toxins) out of your blood and converting them into an intermediary metabolite. This happens by using certain vitamins, minerals, and nutrients like b-vitamins, vitamin c, vitamin E, and others

This phase is easier for your liver to handle since if you're taking a good activated multi-vitamin or eating a high quality and varied diet you are most likely getting these nutrients on a daily basis.

PHASE 2 DETOX

Phase 2 detox is when sulfur based nutrients like n-acetyl cysteine, glutathione, and other nutrients such as glutamine and glycine are needed to change the intermediary metabolite into a harmless water-soluble molecule that can be safely excreted through your urine, stool, or sweat.

Phase 2 detox is typically where we see a breakdown in the body's ability to convert the intermediary metabolites to water soluble waste during this step. Your liver simply lacks the raw material it needs to complete the process at the same rate as the demand placed upon it

Therefore, when someone lacks these phase 2 nutrients which are not common in multi-vitamins or the standard diet, they cannot fully remove toxins. This means your liver then recirculates these toxins back into the blood where they can cause damage or be stored in the brain or bodily tissues. All of this leads to an accumulation of toxins and total toxic load. It is the reason why the *Rain Barrel Effect* is the answer we've been missing.

It's also worth noting that supplementation alone is not enough. This is why specific foods and diet plans are used to cut down on the amount of toxins coming in. Additionally, keeping the bowels moving, sweating, resting, reducing stress, and potentially adding in intestinal cleanses and liver detoxes can be helpful in your detoxification process.

THE FINAL FACTOR

If you truly want to *Empty Your Rain Barrel*™ and heal faster than you ever thought possible, fasting of some type must enter the equation. *(In the next part of this book, I explain which type is best for whom, but for now I want you to know the principles behind it.)*

Fasting has been written about since the dawn of time. It is included in every major religion and every form of medicine except the conventional medicine of today. It is hands down one of the most important "treatments" you can use to allow your body to heal itself.

Fasting is simply a period of time where you do not eat. Drinking water or herbal tea is permitted, but no food can be consumed. This allows the body to rest since it will not have to use any energy for digestion, which can divert up to 30% of all your energy each day to the task of breaking down food. The other thing fasting does is keep your body (and blood) from allowing any new food based toxins in.

Since food based toxins make up the majority of all toxins, this gives your body a tremendous boost in internal energy from not having to work on new incoming chemicals. Remember, even healthy foods have toxic byproducts from their metabolic breakdown, so by not eating for a period of time your total toxic load is lessened.

The act of fasting then allows for your liver to process what you currently have floating around in your blood. You can actually see this principle at work everywhere in nature. If you have a dog or pet, you'll notice that it naturally knows to stop eating when it doesn't feel well. In Ayurvedic Medicine, they knew the healing power of fasting 6,000 years ago and it is a cornerstone of each healing protocol.

NOBEL PRIZE WINNING DISCOVERY

In 2016, The Nobel Prize in Medicine was given to Dr. Yoshinori Ohsumi for his research into *Autophagy*. This discovery was what Functional Medicine and all ancient forms of healing were looking for to prove the efficacy of fasting.

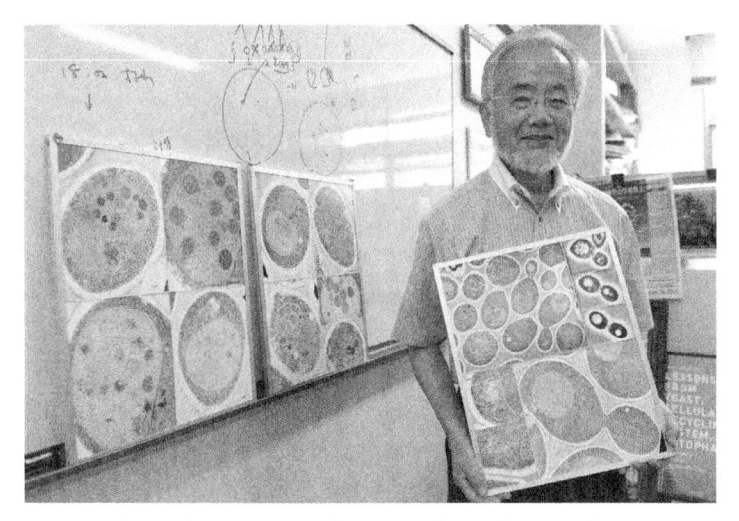

(Dr. Ohsumi's research on autophagy that won him the prestigious Nobel Prize in Medicine.)

Autophagy is the process that takes place in the body during a fasted state. What happens is that when your body does not have any new toxins coming in, it begins to look for new food and fuel sources, as well as to "clean house." This means that your immune system begins to literally eat up dead diseased tissue and kill pathogens in your body.

The new scientific evidence now explains how fasting has been used throughout the world since the beginning of time to aid the body's own natural healing processes. Remember, as advanced as we believe we are in medicine, we still cannot match our innate healing ability. As a Naturopath and Functional Medicine practitioner, my job is to simply give the body what it needs in a supportive capacity and then allow it to heal itself.

One one of the best analogies I can make when describing autophagy is by referring to the old video game, "PAC-MAN." In PAC-MAN a little cartoon head moves around the maze eating up all sorts of "pellets."

You can think of your body as containing its own "PAC-MEN" and when you complete a fast you allow less of the pellets (toxins) to come in, and therefore, your PAC-MEN can gobble up the existing toxic pellets inside you faster.

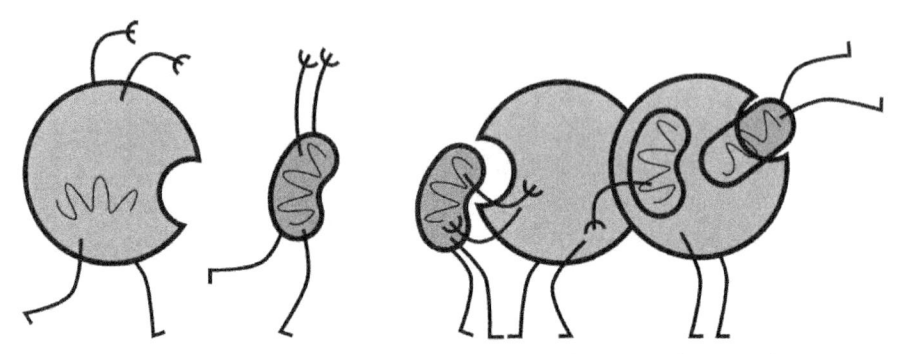

(Here's an immune system PAC-MAN photo of this autophagy analogy eating up all the toxins floating around in your blood.)

Also, please keep in mind that although fasting or any of the d etox methods mentioned may be brand new to you, they have been practiced longer than any other form of medicine in the world and many clinics have brought ancient Ayurvedic treatments to a state-of-the-art level. Not to mention, they simply magnify your body's own healing systems.

21ST CENTURY AYURVEDA

World renowned clinics like the Gerson Institute, founded by Dr. Max Gerson, use (liver based) detoxification as their primary therapy to help cancer patients get well again. These clinics and many others all around the world found the secret to getting well. They know how to integrate the best of ancient healing practices with advanced medical technology.

I didn't know it at the time, but when Dr. Peet was helping me get well, she was doing so by recommending specific foods, rest, and nutritional supplements to give my body what it was missing in order to detox and heal.

Beyond the cortisol, gut and histamine imbalances I suffered from, a few other specific detox issues I had to contend with were genetic MTHFR, and other COMT detox based gene mutations (which are more common than you'd think). It wasn't until I started supporting these genetic issues that I could more fully heal.

During my healing process, Dr. Peet went on to explain to me how having a background in Ayurvedic and Naturopathic Medicine should be my foundation, but that I should accompany that with Functional Medicine. She believed the Ayurvedic Vaidyas (doctors) would have used Functional Medicine had it been around thousands of years ago.

Functional Medicine simply put is the integration of all forms of medicine that work on a holistic (whole health) level. Unlike conventional medicine, Functional Medicine practitioners use their knowledge of "modern medicine," but also look for the underlying root cause of why someone is not well or can't lose weight.

Finding Functional Medicine and advanced lab testing that looks for the hidden, underlying root causes is finally where I found my home in practicing natural health. I could finally combine my love for state-of-the-art science and research with traditional naturopathy and ancient healing wisdom. It's literally the best of both worlds and the DESTRESS Protocol™ that I teach other practitioners and my private wellness clients alike, is the culmination of what I've discovered.

(You will get this exact protocol for getting well, losing weight, and renewing your entire body and mind in Part 4.)

THE FOUNTAIN OF YOUTH REDISCOVERED

At many of the clinics I interned at overseas, I saw hundreds of healthy people walk in as well. At first, I didn't understand why healthy people were coming to a place where sick people came to get well.

I was young and naive to the fact that if you want to stay well, you must continue to do the things that got you healthy. You have to keep detoxifying the body with proven methods, not just wait until you become sick, overweight, or run down.

This was another eye-opening moment for me. I remembered reading in my Ayurvedic textbooks how every season a detox was completed and then at least 1-2x a year, yogis and other healers would go through Pancha Karma treatments themselves to stay healthy and live longer.

We know now that these detoxification treatments helped to purify their body (and mind) and keep them more youthful. This is also why I now preach the benefits and importance of getting well, and then continuing to follow a healthy protocol like the one you're about to receive next. More than ever, it's crucial to support your body on a daily basis and then a few times a year (seasonally if you choose) complete a deeper detoxification protocol.

Now, before we get to the actual DESTRESS Protocol™ for you to learn how to Empty Your Rain Barrel™, I want to share with you one of my favorite science experiment stories that should help to clarify and solidify the need for keeping your body's blood and internal workings pure...

THE IMMORTAL CHICKEN HEART

One of the best examples of how vital it is to keep your blood and cells clean is that of an experiment conducted in 1912, when a group of researchers at Rockefeller Institute in New York City were studying how to keep chicken heart tissue alive on a glass slide.

Amazingly, the living chicken heart tissue continued to pulse day in and day out. However, the trick was that in order to keep the heart alive and in good health, the liquid surrounding the heart had to be changed daily.

This same experiment was kept going for 34 years and the heart kept on pumping even though the average life span for a chicken is only 14 years! And the only reason the heart stopped pumping was that the 3rd generation of scientists no longer wanted to keep up with the experiment and change the heart's solution daily – *not because it died.*

This study also raised some interesting moral questions. What if cellular aging could be eliminated or reversed based on its terrain or solution?

Meaning, if your cells were always bathing in pristine blood and its interstitial milieu (the fluid that feeds the cells and takes out the waste) were kept pure and clean would cellular and biological aging cease?

It's an interesting theory, which needs to be explored to a much greater degree. For now, it's best we don't wait for the decades of scientific research it will take to prove this. We can cleanse the blood, detoxify the body, and prevent disease today.[5]

THE NEXT STEP

I hope by now I've been able to demonstrate the vital importance of lowering your total toxic load and body burden.

It is no longer an option to ignore the environmental, cosmetic, and food based toxins that surround us in this unhealthy world. We must take back our health and our environment. The best way to do that is to Empty Your Rain Barrel™ to remove what you've currently accumulated over the past few decades

It is with great pleasure that I'd now like to teach you exactly how to combine those 6,000 year old Ayurvedic secrets with state-of-the-art science. I call this method my DESTRESS Protocol™. It is quite simply a step-by-step plan that will allow you to finally get well, lose the weight, and feel alive again.

Now let's get started!

Part 4
The DESTRESS Protocol

Diet

Have you ever noticed the insane amount of diet books to choose from? It literally seems like every day there's a new fad diet being hyped by the media. One day it's low carb/high-protein, another day it's high carb/low fat, and the next it's high fat, low carb and low protein.

It's no wonder people are so confused. It's easy to understand why they might just throw their hands up in the air and give up.

That's why in my practice, I teach people *how* to eat. By this I mean, I help them to understand how their body works, which foods cause the most allergies or sensitives, and why all this matters.

Plus, I typically start everyone out with my elimination diet. I researched this elimination diet extensively, after tedious research on the most common autoimmune and gut-triggering inflammatory foods. This allows me to help thousands of people without having to further fine-tune their diets to eliminate things like nightshades, salicylates, high-lectin, or histamine foods.

For the first time ever, I'm going to share this diet plan with you, so that you too can begin to experience the same great results as if you were a private client in my practice.

I really do want you to begin enjoying life and food again, and my straightforward food plan will help you do just that!

ALL THE BEST DIETS ARE THE SAME

There seems to be a lot of controversy over nothing.

I know that when you read a Paleo, Primal, Mediterranean, Vegan, Vegetarian, Pescatarian, Lacto-Ovo Vegetarian, etc., diet book they seem to be taking a new, completely different approach to health and weight loss.

But they're really not.

When you look at good diet books by nutritionists and health practitioners, they are all pretty much saying the same thing.

Out of the thousand or so books on different diet and food healing approaches that I've researched, ones by reputable health writers and nutritionists, I feel confident in telling you that all of the best diets are 80% the same . . .

And what are those similarities?

VEGETABLES

They all recommend vegetables as the main food group and the majority of the diet. This means that for most true-health diets, about two-thirds of each meal or total food intake should be vegetables.

This equates to a diet of 60-70% vegetables.

FRUIT

Next up we have fruit. Some diets recommend quite a bit of fruit, but most strive for 2-4 servings per day. The fruit should mostly be lower fructose and lower glycemic (I'll provide a list in a moment).

Now some diets do cut fruit out in the beginning, but typically they allow it to be reintroduced slowly after a 1-3 week elimination.

I use this same protocol and my clients have achieved exceptional body transformation results with this approach to fruits.

FATS

So now that we have about 70% of the diet locked up with vegetables and fruit, there's only a maximum of 30% left. And, every diet, even a low fat one, recommends at least 10-20% fat as part of your macronutrient ratio. (Macronutrients are measured in grams or calories from fats, carbohydrates, and proteins.)

Of course, ketogenic diets recommend a much higher fat intake, but these are short-sighted and completely neglect the importance of many fruits, vegetables and carbs that are crucial for health.

PROTEINS

It's the one food group that is causing more battles, bickering, and points of contention than any other group. But, when you look at my breakdown you'll begin to see what I saw…

When I give seminars, I show this visual and pie graph. I don't like food pyramids because they give you a diagram that implies one food is more important than another.

That's simply not the case. For optimal healthy living and longevity, we need all the food groups listed above. If we don't get them, our bodies and mind begin to suffer. That's why I don't advocate any diet that goes too heavy on any one macronutrient to the detriment of another.

VEGAN, VEGETARIAN OR MEAT EATER

First, let's briefly define these groups.

Vegans believe in the humane treatment of animals and that non-animal based products should be our primary source of nutrition, and therefore, do not eat anything that comes from animal sources (meat, fish, eggs, dairy, honey, etc.).

Vegetarians may eat fish, dairy or eggs, but they will not eat meat. Both groups often times also point to research showing an animal-based diet can increase health risks.

Meat eaters will quickly point out that it is processed carbohydrates that increase health risks, and not good quality meat.

So, who's right?

The truth is they *both can be* right and it honestly doesn't matter all that much (in terms of long-term health) when you're using my food circle.

The reason for this is that no matter if you're eating fish, eggs, meat, or a plant based protein, only about 10-15% of your diet is going to be protein. So in the grand scheme of things that small amount will most likely have a much smaller effect on your health.

Please also keep in mind that the 10-20% macronutrient ratio for protein in your diet is also in direct alignment with the best research on the longest-lived cultures all across the world, as revealed in the *Blue Zones*.

PALEO SHOCK WAVES

For hardcore paleo advocates this may come as a shock. I believe in the "Paleo diet" for the most part – just not what it's morphed into.

No Paleolithic human ever had the option or ability to eat meat 3-5x a day 365-days of the year. It's an insane concept, which will lead to poor health after years of following it. The unfortunate part is that it's often the slow accumulation of illness, which prevents people from ever seeing it coming.

For example, many Paleo followers may eat bacon, eggs, and avocado for breakfast, a grass-fed burger or chicken sausage for lunch, and a piece of salmon for dinner – and maybe snack on some beef jerky mid-day. Does that look anything like what a hunter-gatherer, forager, or Paleo man would eat?

There's no chance.

Just for a moment, picture yourself in the wild. What would you be eating? How would you have access to a solely meat-based breakfast? Have you ever thought about how hard it would be to catch and kill a 4-legged animal with your bare hands, a rock, or a spear? And before fire was "invented" don't you think it may be difficult to bite through an animal's hide, then chew and swallow all that animal muscle without cooking it?

Wouldn't it be more plausible that you'd hunt and gather during the day and then eat what you caught (if anything) that afternoon or evening? Wouldn't that be more "Paleo?"

I pose these questions not to be confrontational, but simply as points to reflect upon. My goal is to simply expand your mind and get you to see that there doesn't need to be one dogmatic form of thought.

(Note: This chapter and the others to follow in the DESTRESS Protocol™ could all fill their own 300-page book. Therefore, I cannot breakdown every topic in depth. However, my intention with this book was never to give you every extraneous detail, but rather a foundation to build on – which by the way is all most people will ever need. On the resource page I will detail more in depth diet plans, exercise programs, etc.)

A RETURN TO COMMON SENSE EATING

To be honest, eating healthy often times just comes back to common sense. The problem is that we've been brainwashed by the media.

There's no other way to describe these strange new inventions in diet approaches. It boggles my mind that anyone would think eating a solely fat-based diet is key to nutrition. How could you possibly get your vitamin C that way? And what about the fiber and carbohydrates needed to feed your healthy gut microbiome (intestinal bacteria).

Although many keto devotees say they advocate eating vegetables, when you look at what they're really eating to lean down – you'll notice most of them consume a diet based on virtually all fats. Fat doesn't spike insulin, they argue, helping you run on your own fat for fuel.

But where are the antioxidants? Where are the vitamins? Where are the phytonutrients we need for just basic health? What I'm recommending is a return to health and a plan to reduce the toxic overload from the foods we are eating.

Therefore, I'm not going to tell you to be a vegan, vegetarian, or meat eater, what I am saying is that a natural human diet across the board should look virtually the same with the exception of about 4-8oz of fish, egg, animal, or vegan protein per day.

POWERFUL DIET FACTORS

Besides looking at the macronutrient profile of your diet – that is, how much of your diet is made up of fats, protein, starches, fruits, and vegetables – there are powerful factors that can literally turn hormones on and off and affect your genetic code. These factors dictate your health, longevity, and body shape.

So before we get into the detoxifying diet and how to Empty Your Rain Barrel™ through food, let's review the often overlooked details about nutrition that have just as much of an effect on health as what you eat.

WHEN TO EAT

You may remember earlier when I spoke of the Nobel-Prize winning research on autophagy that this process takes place when we're *not* eating...

As discussed earlier, we call this intermittent fasting (IF) and it's been used in every form of natural medicine since the dawn of time. It's something we even see animals use when they're not feeling well – they just stop eating until they get well.

But did you know there are also natural rhythms to eating? Eating that flows with the seasons and the time of day we consume foods, for example.

Our bodies are intimately synced up to our environment and the cycles of the sun and moon and following these clues in nature can help you live a healthier life.

For example, as the sun rises each day, our bodies switch from an overnight detoxifying and repair mode (anabolism) to a more catabolic state during the day. The same process is seen in nature as flowers open with sunlight during the day and close up with the moon at night.

Believe it or not, we're intimately connected to nature. After all, we've only been living in homes with electricity for just a few hundred years.

Our bodies were built to burn up food during the day and then "clean house" at night when it's dark and there's no work to be done. That's why we are meant to rest at night and our circadian rhythms fight this in every way if we don't. So, it's pretty easy to see when you should be eating.

YOUR WINDOW TO EAT

Some people say, don't eat after 5, or 7, or 9, but what they're all trying to say is, don't eat late at night… It makes sense and it's backed up both by science and 6,000+ years of Ayurvedic teaching.

The best time for consuming food is from about 6:00/7:00AM – 6:00/7:00PM. Times may vary based on the seasons, but there is no need to make it more complicated than this.

COMPLETE A DAILY 12-HOUR FAST

So judging from the example above, you can now see why intermittent fasting has become so popular and rightly so. The research on it now is undeniable.

Whenever I mention a daily 12-hour fast in my practice the first thought many people have is "how would that ever be possible?" This thought is then quickly followed up by, "won't I be starving?"

The answer to these questions and many others is actually simpler than you may think. To complete a daily 12-hour fast, all you must do is stop eating after dinner. That's it. If you stop eating at 7:00pm, go to bed around 10:00pm, sleep until 6:00am, and then have breakfast at 7:00am, you just completed a 12-hour fast.

Honestly, it is that easy and the results will astound you!

Just from this tip alone I've seen people lose the weight, improve their digestion, increase energy, and eliminate brain fog. Much of this comes from allowing the body to get back into a rhythm of eating when the body does its best job breaking down food and then allowing for natural elimination and detoxification at night.

This is most effective when you go to bed with a near empty stomach and this can only be achieved when you stop eating 2-3 hours before bed. Doing so allows your stomach to rest and move most of its food contents into the small intestine where further breakdown can take place. Then your body can shift its state to one of relaxation and repair overnight instead of keeping energy high for digestion.

Inevitably, someone will bring up the benefits of having a small snack before bed. However, this is only recommended when someone is suffering from adrenal fatigue and cannot properly balance their low blood sugar levels.

For these people, I do agree with a small snack before bed and I would allow a small protein/fat snack 30-minutes prior to sleep. The caveat to this is that the end goal should eventually be to achieve this 12-hour fast once you rebalance your body and recover from your adrenal fatigue (which can be attained within 12-16 weeks for most people).

The bottom line is that you must respect your body's natural rhythms of when to eat and when not to eat. If you don't, it will send you the symptoms of dis-ease such as poor health, weight gain, brain fog, dull skin, disrupted sleep, and fatigue.

But now that you know how easy it is to do, you can complete a 12-hour fast with ease!

LIQUID BEFORE LUNCH

The next concept is something I developed in my practice a number of years ago. It's only been in the past 4-5 years, though, that I've realized how powerful it is.

Although I certainly did not invent the "no whole food before lunch" concept, I believe I've pushed it forward by coming up with a happy medium.

By this I mean there are many people that advocate a longer fast from around dinner time (7:00pm) to lunch the next day (12:00pm). This equates to a 15-16 hour fast. They believe that longer fasts lead to more detoxification. And I can't disagree with that.

But what I *can* disagree with is that it's not necessarily healthy for most people to fast that long on a daily basis.

The reason for this is once you begin to come under pressure from the day (think work stress, rush hour traffic, or getting kids ready in the morning), your body is going start producing larger amounts of norepinephrine and cortisol. Fasting only causes more stress on your body and exacerbates that stress hormone release.

At this point your body is going to look to combat this stress with a short-term fuel source like glucose (sugar). If it's not there, it may tap into muscle stores. This stress hormone cycle eventually leads to a weakened metabolism, low thyroid, lowered sex hormones, and low immune system. It's certainly not ideal.

That's why I recommend most people eat breakfast, but keep it light. This typically means having a glass of water with lemon, lime, or greens powder to wake up your digestive system and then about 60-90 minutes after waking you can enjoy a fresh pressed vegetable juice or ideally, an all-in-one smoothie for breakfast.

A SMOOTHIE A DAY

It's quite possible that no one loves smoothies more than I do.

This is because I realized many years ago when I was on my path to getting well that my digestive system was so weak from eating poorly that almost any food would make me bloated or cause some fatigue. I actually felt best when I didn't eat!

Although it's not normal to feel bloating, indigestion, or fatigue after eating, digesting food does take an enormous amount of energy. The statistics state about 30% of all of your energy for the day goes to breaking down the food you eat.

Plus, if you have a weakened digestive system, which many people unknowingly do, you can imagine how much more energy would be needed to break down each meal . . .

This is why when I realized that easy-to-digest foods would require less digestive energy, leaving more energy for me, I began drinking smoothies (blended shakes) multiple times per day. After only about 2-3 weeks of testing out this theory I had already begun to get my energy back.

It was nothing short of amazing.

Now I recommend a smoothie for breakfast to all my clients because I know it will be the #1 thing they can do for their body in terms of diet. An AM smoothie will draw very little digestive energy from your body and will provide more nutrition than you could most likely absorb from a whole food meal.

However, the smoothies really are whole food meals in blended format. There's not a lot of mystery to them. They are a meal with carbs, protein, and fat all mixed together. *(Although there is much merit to food combining, when you blend all foods up to a liquid consistency most individuals tolerate it exceptionally well.)*

These smoothies will allow you to keep more of your own energy for other metabolic processes – which in turn leads to stabilizing and enhancing your mood, clearer thinking, heightened energy, and feeling more alive!

HOW TO MAKE A SMOOTHIE

I'll provide my personal daily smoothie recipe in the back appendix of the book, but to make the concept easier to imagine, I blend:

- 16-20 oz. of water (or substitute 8oz nut milk)
- 1-2 cups of a low glycemic fruit
- 1-2 cups of green leafy veggies (or greens powder)
- 2 scoops all-in-one protein powder (includes a full methylated/activated multi-vitamin with 100%+ of the RDA of vitamins for the day)
- Optional add-ons can include 1TBSP of flax or chia seeds and coconut oil for a health fat

One caveat: For those just starting out, I never recommend adding in the green leafy vegetables, seeds, or extra fat in the beginning. The reason is that even though it is blended and broken down, it can still be too hard to digest for weaker digestive systems. It's best to simply start with just a cup of berries, water (or an unsweetened nut milk), and the all-in-one powder (which includes fiber).

AM DETOX

The other benefit to waking up with some warm water and lemon and a smoothie is that they hydrate every cell in your body. The truth is that many people are chronically dehydrated and that's also why drinking a smoothie for breakfast can be life-changing. The joint pain, inflammation, headaches, congestion, and fatigue are often a manifestation of this cellular dehydration and the only cure is more water – especially when it's loaded with minerals.

And finally, the last reason why a smoothie is the #1 breakfast in the morning is because it allows you to flush the toxins from your body that had accumulated overnight while sleeping. The natural stagnation state of lying down must be balanced with a clearing out each morning (more on this later).

If you're not already drinking a smoothie every morning, this easy, low cost breakfast will provide all the fuel you need before lunch. If you do nothing else, this is my highest recommendation for improving your health, reshaping your body, and waking up your brain.

COFFEE & CAFFEINE

The powerful breakfast smoothie I mentioned above is loaded with antioxidants and will jumpstart the detoxification process each morning. Truthfully, I think you'll find very little need for coffee or caffeine once you begin your day with a smoothie.

Coffee has become a crutch to wake us up and get us through the day. If this is the case with you, I'd take a good hard look at that. If you need artificial stimulants to give you an energy boost, something is wrong in your body. You're not producing your own natural energy and therefore you need to kick start it with caffeine.

The other issue is that caffeine also slows the detoxification process. So, my recommendation is to follow my caffeine weaning protocol, which allows you to cut back to just one small cup in the morning (or completely eliminate it).

HOW TO WEAN OFF CAFFEINE

- Week 1: Make the same size coffee, but use ½ decaf
- Week 2: Move down 1 size coffee and stay with ½ decaf
- Week 3: Move to just a small coffee, ½ decaf, or all decaf
- Week 4: Maintain with a small coffee or switch to green or herbal tea

(Note: Decaf coffee should be organic, Swiss water processed to avoid toxins.)

I've given this protocol to thousands of people to wean off all types of caffeine without the headaches and withdrawal symptoms and I know it will work for you too.

I'll be talking more about energy balance, exercise, and the adrenal glands later in this book, but please do keep in mind that just because a food or beverage is enjoyable doesn't mean we need to rationalize why it's good for us. This happens with alcohol and coffee far more than it should…

Now, I do understand that you may just love the taste of coffee and if that's the case I simply ask that you use an organic blend and keep it to one cup before 1:00pm every day. The organic varieties will keep you from swallowing larger amounts of pesticides and having caffeine before 1:00 pm works best with the natural cortisol rhythms of your body.

FOUNDATIONAL FOODS

Now that we have a few of the diet basics covered, let's go over the foods I recommend starting out with as you're trying to lower your total toxic load and Empty Your Rain Barrel™.

WATER

Although I mentioned that the foundation of every diet should start with vegetables, what I didn't mention was that water is just as crucial. Our bodies are made of approximately 2/3rds water and even going one day without it can begin to harm our physiology.

Ideally, though, we're looking for the water you consume to be pure spring water or filtered. Tap water is just too contaminated with pharmaceutical drugs, heavy metals like aluminum, as well as fluoride and chlorine. All of these slowly weaken your immune system, deteriorate your nervous system, and fill up your rain barrel.

On the resource page for this book I give a more in depth breakdown and provide a range of water filters for every budget. And, on Instagram.com/stephencabral I also have dozens of posts on this topic and many more.

On a daily basis, your goal should be to drink about half your body weight (lbs.) in water (oz.) per day. For example, if you weigh 160 lbs., then you would aim for 80oz. of water, which is 10 glasses per day. Please keep in mind that your smoothie, lemon water, greens drink, vegetable juice, and herbal tea *do count* towards your total water consumption. Although this is a close approximation, some people may need more (or less) depending on other lifestyle and health factors.

PROTEIN LIST

Again, without writing an entire book on just a diet plan, the best way to look at proteins is to begin to view this food group in a whole new light.

I used to center every one of my meals around a big slab of protein. I was obsessed with building a bigger and stronger body. What I didn't realize was all that meat and protein was hurting me internally. I was constantly tired, bloated, and catching every cold from overconsuming protein to the count of over 200 grams per day.

It's important to keep in mind that most factory-farmed animals live in deplorable and unsanitary conditions where they are exposed to sickness, stress, disease, and filth. They're also fed GMO corn, soy, and other grains that their bodies were never meant to eat. As a result, they get sick. So as a preemptive measure to this disease state, most cattle feed is laced with antibiotics – so much so that now more than 60% all antibiotics in the United States are given to cattle – not prescribed to people![1]

Unless you're purchasing pasture-raised chickens, grass-fed and finished beef, or wild fish, you're most likely doing more harm than good for your body.

Eating fish now is not much better. The seas have been polluted with toxic waste, plastics and other chemicals that all make their way into the seafood we consume. The oceans have been overfished and we're now resorting to "farm-raising" many varieties of fish, crustacean, and mollusks. However, don't let the cute name fool you. Fish are grown in tanks or plastic swimming pools with unclean water conditions where they swim in their own feces and are fed the same grains and antibiotics as our cattle.[2]

It's sad to see how low we've sunk. What's worse is that most people don't even know that this is going on. To find out more about these issues, I recommend watching documentaries like *Food Inc.* and others. I provide a fully updated recommendation list on my resource page.

Although I believe we should all be doing our part in the long-run to boycott this treatment of animals, destruction of the earth (methane gas and waste runoff), and perversion of our food sources, I think there's a quicker fix that's more realistic for most people in the long-run.

All we have to do is cut way back on the amount of animal products we consume. If you're a big animal protein eater, cut back to just a handful at lunch and dinner. Or, better yet just have meat or fish at one meal per day only. Then you can add in some non-meat days eventually. What seems difficult now becomes very easy in just a matter of weeks...

Here are healthier protein options to choose from:

Animal (pastured or grass-fed)

- Chicken
- Turkey
- Duck
- Game meat
- Organ meat

- Eggs
- Lamb
- Buffalo

Fish (wild, low mercury)

- Salmon
- Trout
- Sea bass
- Sardines
- Anchovies
- Mackerel
- Shrimp
- Cod
- Haddock

Vegan

- Chickpeas
- Beans of all type (not canned baked beans)
- Quinoa
- Non-GMO organic sprouted tofu (1-2x a week if non-estrogen dominant)
- Lentils
- Split mung beans
- Hemp hearts
- Sprouts
- Rice & pea protein powder

FAT LIST

Fat is vital for our mood, brain, organs, nervous system, and energy, but it's crucial we stay balanced and choose the right fats.

When I look at advanced genetic testing on how much each "allele" or different genotype (body-type) should take in for fat, it varies between 10 – 35%.

That's why although I do recommend genetic testing to know more about your body, most people should aim to stay around 15-30% maximum from this macronutrient.

The genetic research goes even deeper and it shows that if you are a 4-allele APOe genotype you're not going to do as well with saturated fat.[3] For these types of genotypes, eating too much saturated fat will cause more inflammation. It's also why I cringe anytime I see all these keto-diet recommendations as an all-for-one approach. It's dangerous advice for many, since 26% of the population carries this 4 allele!

The healthiest fats will always come from whole foods and since you now know you'll be cutting back on your meat consumption, you'll be getting most of your fats from these foods:

- Avocado
- Coconut *(does contain forms of saturated fat)*
- Olives
- Seeds
- Nuts

If you're using oils such as coconut and olive oil, do make sure to get 100% organic, extra-virgin, first and cold pressed to ensure it is top quality without additives.

My other recommendation to cut back on oxidation and inflammation in your body is to use your olive oil or other oils as a dressing instead of cooking with them. This prevents their delicate molecular structure from breaking down under heat. Even acceptable high heat fats like coconut oil, grass-fed butter, or ghee are best used on a low heat or as a dressing after the food has been served.

VEGETABLE LIST

As humans, we are uniquely suited to consume plenty of vegetables and they should make up the majority of our diet. They are mineral rich and loaded with anti-cancer phytonutrients.

Plus, the majority of our fiber each day will come mainly from vegetables if we're eating enough. This will allow for numerous cardiovascular and digestive benefits. Ideally, women will aim for at least 35g a day in fiber, and men should shoot for 40g.

The easiest way to keep up with your vegetables is to simply look to include 1-2 cups minimum, per meal. They can be raw, cooked, or blended depending on your preference and the season. For example, if your digestion is weak, it's best to cook your food and allow the heat to predigest the cellulose plant structure. This will enable your digestive system to have to do less work and you'll absorb more nutrients.

Also, if it's winter and you live in a cold climate like I do in Boston, you may not want to eat a lot of salads. This time of the year, you may prefer cooked spinach or other warm vegetables instead and save your raw foods for the Spring and Summer (as Ayurveda teaches us).

Here is a list of vegetables to choose from:

- Spinach
- Kale
- Chard
- Romaine
- Mustard greens
- Arugula

- Parsnips
- Heirloom tomatoes
- Cucumber
- Celery
- Bok choy
- Sprouts
- Bamboo shoots
- Endive
- Brussels sprouts
- Turnips
- Carrots
- Snap peas
- Green beans
- Parsnips
- Beets
- Asparagus
- Broccoli
- Cauliflower
- Radishe

Remember, vegetables are the very best way we can detoxify our body using whole foods and that's why we must make sure to include a rainbow of colors each day in our diet!

GLUTEN-FREE STARCH LIST

Starches are often a source of debate among experts, due to their unwillingness to stay open to the fact that different people require varied levels of carbohydrates.

Ayurvedic Medicine has known for thousands of years that the Vata body type (ectomorph) needs more carbohydrates to decrease cortisol, keep up with energy demands, and calm the central nervous system. It's also why low-carb diets are crippling for this body type. However, the Kapha body type (endomorph) does well with less starch and a lower daily carbohydrate total coming mainly from vegetables.

Regardless of body type, each individual can do well with some form of a gluten-free starch as long as they are active. The amount will vary depending on energy, metabolism, hormone, and weight loss goals. If you're looking to lose weight it may be best to keep your serving to just ½ cup at lunch and dinner, or just at lunch until you reach your weight loss goals.

Here is a list of low-inflammatory starches:

Root Vegetables

- Yams, Japanese yams
- Sweet potatoes
- Yucca

Gluten-Free Grains

- Oats
- Rice
- Quinoa
- Amaranth
- Millet
- Buckwheat

FRUIT LIST

Fruit is easily the most misunderstood health food.

We're told it makes us fat, raises our blood sugar, and causes hormone disruption, but this simply isn't true. Fruit can exacerbate all of the above stated conditions, but it isn't the cause. An imbalanced body that can't metabolize sugar at a cellular level is the real issue.[4]

Actually, scientists have determined that much of the cause of heart disease is from inflammation caused by a wide range of factors including dietary toxins, environmental toxins, a high Omega 6 to Omega 3 fat ratio, and a high refined carbohydrate and sugar diet - not a diet high in fruits, vegetable, fiber, and healthy fats![5]

Having said that, for many people on a healing protocol or looking to lose weight, you may want to eliminate fruit or limit your consumption to just berries for the first few weeks before introducing other types. This will give your body time to re-regulate its metabolic processes while emptying your rain barrel of the current sugar load on your body.

After this removal period is over, here are a handful of the healing fruits that are loaded with vitamins, minerals, and anti-cancer compounds (anthocyanins) that you can add back into your diet:

Lower Glycemic

- Blueberries
- Blackberries
- Raspberries
- Cherries
- Strawberries
- Kiwi
- Green Apple

Moderate Glycemic

- Apples
- Oranges
- Grapefruit

Higher Glycemic

- Watermelon
- Mangos
- Papaya (non-GMO)
- Pineapple
- Bananas

FINAL NOTES

In the last part of this book I'll be providing you with the exact 21-day protocol I use for detoxification and diet in my practice, but for now, I'd like to leave you with a sample meal plan that puts it all together for you.

THE EMPTY YOUR RAIN BARREL™ MEAL (DIET) PLAN

As I stated at the very beginning of this chapter, all human diets should have the same core ingredients – healthy fats, vegetables and fruit, a clean source of protein, little to no processed foods, and lots of water!

So here are my top recommendations to ensure you are keeping your toxin levels low and emptying your rain barrel at the same time!

- Eat mostly whole foods – as you would see growing in nature
- Consume very little, if any, boxed, bagged or processed foods
- 60-80% of your diet should be plant based (vegetables & fruits)
- If you eat meat and fish, it should be pastured, grass-fed, or wild
- Your fruits & vegetables should be organic, especially the dirty dozen
- Try not to fry your foods in oil (add your oil after as a dressing)
- Drink ½ your bodyweight in ounces of water each day
- Start your day with an easy to digest breakfast
- Aim for a smoothie to start your day!

Exercise

Where did we go wrong?

Just like the diet fads and crazes we see promoted in the media, we have that same hype-machine working with exercise. One day Pilates is best; then HIIT; then Tabata; then…

Most people are confused as to what to do and after more than 250,000 client appointments, what I see is that most people fall into 1 of the following 3 categories:

1. SEDENTARY

This group is easy to describe because they are not currently exercising. They may consider themselves active, but no weight training or cardiovascular exercise is happening on a daily or even weekly basis. They either tell themselves they do not have the time or they simply abhor the thought of working out.

2. CARDIO ONLY

This group is following well-intentioned, but outdated recommendations from over 40 years ago that suggested long distance cardio and running is what's best for health.

The problem is that long-distance, endurance-based training has now been proven to cause microscopic tears in the heart leading to potential cardiac issues.[1] It's also one of the reasons why marathoners often die at a younger age, despite their "healthy" lifestyle.[2]

3. HARDCORE WORKOUTS

This last group follows the mentality that if a little is good, a lot must be better, and if a lot must be better, then crushing your body with each workout makes it the ultimate way to exercise.

The problem is that working out this hard causes even greater stress on the body and can raise cortisol, inflammation, and blood sugar levels as a response to that trauma. I, too, once believed in this level of exercise.

WHERE WE WENT WRONG

In a moment, I'll explain the proper way to exercise if you want to enjoy a lifetime of results, but for now let's talk about how we got so far off track, so that we know what to fix in the first place.

It seems to be a forgotten concept that exercise is supposed to mimic natural human movement for what our bodies were meant to do. We were born hunter gathers with the ability to sprint, walk long distances, and use our strength when needed to fight, throw objects, or build things.

However, the human body is also designed to conserve energy and not over exert itself due to increased caloric and metabolic demands. This is also true for most mammals. Knowing this, we can now extrapolate all the information we need to create workout programs built for how our bodies were meant to move.

This means that if humans were given a powerful Achilles tendon and large glutes (the largest muscles in your body) for sprinting short distances, we can begin to see how running *long* distances may not be such a good idea.

And, if we're overexerting ourselves with long, strenuous workouts that never include periodic lighter weeks, our bodies are going to break down and get injured. You also run the risk of increasing your blood sugar, inflammation, and hunger levels – potentially leading to added fat weight gain. Since this is the last thing any one wants, it's important we begin to explore why we got into working out in the first place.

HUMBLE BEGINNINGS

20 years ago, I began helping clients transform their bodies through both resistance (weight training) workouts and cardiovascular work. The programs were sound, but they could have been greatly improved.

I used to use a lot more machines with my clients (in the late 90's) and we also did more running than the ideal amount. Around the turn of the new millennium in 2000, "Functional Training" had become more in vogue and those that kept up with the research moved to more natural human movements. This included exercises using mainly free weights like dumbbells, cables, and stability balls.

This is well before the TRX and kettlebell movement became popular, but it was the start to teaching people to value how their body moves naturally versus being forced to do a movement in fixed pattern (like machine circuits at gyms).

Functional movement has now grown to include all types of equipment as long as it allows your body to move naturally, unobstructed, and in an innate range of motion.

ROAD BLOCKS

The only caveat to creating an exercise program that mimics the normal human movement of long distance walking, sprinting, and lifting things (manual labor), is that nature never intended us to sit in our car or at desks for such long periods of time.

Unfortunately, this seated position must be accounted for when designing a workout program to correct the biomechanical deviations (poor posture) created from this much sitting.

For example, your hamstring, hip rotators, and hip flexors need to be lengthened and stretched using specific exercises. If this isn't incorporated into your workout program, you can actually be making them tighter, which is definitely not the goal.

The problem then becomes that this tightness builds up overtime, gradually filling up your rain barrel and can affect your lower back, neck, and ability to move properly. When this happens you begin to compensate and along with that comes pain from being misaligned. Pain also starts a vicious cycle since it can cause you both physical and emotional stress, which elevates your cortisol levels.

This is why realigning your posture and beginning a functional training workout program built to transform your body into the healthy form it was meant to be *is crucial*. Plus, when you begin to exercise, you get many fringe benefits besides just correcting your posture and making you naturally stronger…

Here are the top reasons why exercise will help you Empty Your Rain Barrel™ and improve your wellness, weight loss, and anti-aging goals.

ENDORPHINS

Exercise routinely beats pharmaceutical drugs when they go head to head in trials to see which one better elevates mood and alleviates depression.[3]

If you suffer from high stress, low mood, anxiety, depression, PTSD, panic attacks or other mood disorders, I highly recommend working out almost daily during the morning hours. It very well may just change your life.

METABOLISM

Did you know short bursts of exercise actually improves metabolism over long-distance cardio sessions?[4]

This means you can do interval training that includes 30-90 second sets of exercise with rest periods in between and actually get better results than killing yourself for an hour on the treadmill!

A few examples of intervals are metabolic resistance workouts, Tabatas, spin classes, hill sprints, and stadium stair runs.

Intervals are truly an amazingly efficient way to workout and build your body up rather than breaking it down. I'll provide you with an exact workout for free on my resource page, but here's a snapshot of what a simple, 10-minute interval workout looks like:

- **Warm-Up:** 3-5 minutes of planks, bridging & lunges
- **Interval 1:** Mountain Climbers x 30 seconds
- Rest 30-60 seconds
- **Interval 2:** Frog Jumps x 30 seconds
- Rest 30-60 seconds
- **Interval 3:** Jumping Jacks x 30 seconds
- Rest 30-60 seconds
- **Interval 4:** Speed Skaters x 30 seconds
- Rest 30-60 seconds
- **Interval 5:** Sprinting in Place x 30 seconds
- Done!

(You can download your copy with photos and videos of this workout at StephenCabral.com/rbe)

The best part about the interval above is that you can be any fitness level to complete it and you can do it right at home in just 10-minutes a day!

STILL LOVE CARDIO?

Some people don't want to give up their cardio because of how it makes them feel. To those people I simply recommend not running for more than a couple of miles or keeping it under 30-40 minutes total run time.

After about 40-minutes of training, your cortisol stress hormone levels may begin to rise and your body will actually begin to break down muscle tissue if needed for fuel.

This leads to lower testosterone and a lowered metabolism. It can also negatively impact fitness gains, as well as weaken muscles and bones.

I will say, though, that I have no issues with people enjoying a good run on beautiful day to clear their head and boost endorphins – In the same light, moderate cardio is also an excellent way to oxygenate the tissues and potentially increase telomere length (leading to increased longevity).

RESISTANCE TRAINING

Right now, body weight training is very popular. This is an excellent form of working out where you can still get the stimulus you need to boost your metabolism and strengthen every muscle in your body, as long as you know how to choose your exercises.

I see too many people choosing more chest, bicep, and quad based exercises (beach muscles) and not enough back and glute/hamstring work. By working harder on the muscles like your glutes and hamstrings that may be weaker, you will actually help to rebalance the body. This, in turn, reduces inflammation, alleviates pain, and boosts your mood!

The goal of working out with your own body weight or added resistance is to create change in the body. It's referred to as the SAID Principle and it stands for *Specific Adaptions to Imposed Demands*. This means that you must have a way to challenge the body beyond what it can currently already do.

It's the only way to get your body to change.

Having said that, hardcore boot-camps and 100 rep exercises are not only unnecessary, but they can lead to overuse and repetitive motion injuries.

For detailed workouts please see my *the Rain Barrel Effect's* free resource page or my previously published book, *A Man's Guide to Muscle & Strength* (it's for women too!)

WHERE TO START

If you're not currently completing 10,000 steps of walking per day, this is where to start. To be honest, walking is not exercise – it's activity. It's basic human movement and it must be done on a daily basis.

10,000 steps per day is still about 3,000-8,000 steps less than the estimated amount we humans used to walk a few thousand years ago.

Our bodies were built for this and it's a great way to calm the sympathetic nervous system stress response. Plus, it keeps blood sugar levels regulated and taps into body fat stores.

Getting 10,000 steps a day is also easier than you think.

Three 30-minute walks per day is really all you need. But, it's really even simpler than that since most people at a desk job that I have track their walking in a day (before starting a walking protocol) average about 3,500-4,000 steps per day. This is just from normal walking around and commuting.

The bad news is that means most people are only walking for about 30-40 minutes per day since a typical walking average is 1,000 steps for every

10-minutes walked. But, there is some good news… To reach 10,000 steps per day they only need to add 6,000 more, which is as easy as a lunch-time walk and a post-dinner stroll.

If you have a dog, take them for a nice 30-minute walk. And, if you begin an exercise program, you'll be covered for the additional steps during that workout. Walking is more important than you think to help rebalance your body and keep it strong for life.

Only after you work up to 10,000 steps per day should you really worry about getting into a formal workout program.

WORKING OUT WHILE TIRED

My number one recommendation to everyone I meet with is to never leave a workout with less energy than they came in. Ever.

This means that you must stop when you begin to peak. You'll be feeling great at this point in your workout and it will actually be hard to pull back, since you'll naturally want to use up some of that extra energy you feel. Fight that urge.

This is one of the recommendations I use for chronic fatigue and auto-immune suffers in my practice. And, it just so happens to work amazingly well when followed by others too for general health.

What transpires inside your body is that you leave your workout feeling an endorphin high, which cuts your pain and eases your stress without further burning out your nervous system. Then, your body gets to rebuild from a natural anabolic growth hormone, DHEA, and testosterone standpoint, without the influx of cortisol, which is catabolic and breaks the body down.

This is a powerful and greatly misunderstood biochemical principle and when not overdone, exercise can also help you balance your immune system (Th1/Th2) and get well again.

If you're trying to overcome a particular health issue right now, in the beginning you will only want to exercise every other day. The reason is that working out everyday can cause too large an increase in excitatory neurotransmitters, adrenaline, cortisol, and inflammation, which can hinder your recovery process in the long-term.

By giving yourself a full day off in between workouts you'll recover faster and not over tax your depleted reserves. Plus, this will allow ample time to drop inflammation levels before taxing your muscles and nervous system again.

It's also as simple as choosing a Monday, Wednesday, Friday workout plan that combines both resistance training and/or some intervals or light cardio. As your body gets stronger, you can increase the length, intensity, and the amount of days you exercise. And keep in mind, that you'll still be walking 10,000 steps per day – every day.

(Note: For a complete progression of how to ramp up your workouts from beginner to intermediate to advanced check out my free podcast at: StephenCabral.com/573)

There's plenty of time, so don't rush things. In other words, go easy – this is the only body you were given!

The next chapter will also give you a better idea of how you'll know *when* you can increase your workouts.

EMPTY YOUR RAIN BARREL™ IDEAL WORKOUT WEEK

In a perfect world, this is the ideal week of exercise I'd recommend. It balances soft and hard forms of movement and is perfect for almost anyone that is not competing for a specific goal (bodybuilding, powerlifting, sport specific, etc.). Remember, it's something to strive for even if you can only do half of what's listed!

METHODS OF EXERCISE

Walking Days = 7 (10,000 steps total per day)
Resistance Training Days = 3
Cardio Days = 2
Formal Yoga or Stretching Class = 2

SAMPLE WEEKLY SCHEDULE

Monday: Resistance training workout #1 (may add 3-5 intervals after workout)
Tuesday: Cardio workout #1 (bike, run, row, sprint, etc.)
Wednesday: Resistance training workout #2 (may add 3-5 intervals after workout)
Thursday: Gentle Yoga, Qi Gong, Tai Chi, Stretching Class, or Rest
Friday: Resistance training workout #3 (may add 3-5 intervals after workout)
Saturday: Cardio workout #2 (bike, run, row, sprint, etc.)
Sunday: Gentle Yoga, Qi Gong, Tai Chi, Stretching Class or Rest

NOTES:

- Each workout should be 20-40 minutes in duration
- Stretching should be done 1-2x a day (daily) for 5-10 minutes to stay flexible and calm the sympathetic nervous system

Download the ideal workout week and free online personal training workouts and exercise videos at: StephenCabral.com/rbe

Stress Reduction

Stress is one of those topics that people seem to brush under the rug… They know it's important, but if they give any real thought to it and how it may be affecting their overall health, body, and longevity they may just scare themselves. If you haven't heard yet, stress is the attributed underlying root cause or causal factor in the expression of almost every known dis-ease.

This includes all auto-immune and weight based issues, since the delicate balance of hormones plays such a crucial role in maintaining equilibrium within the body. Remember, your rain barrel overflows when stress reaches its upper limit in your mind and body!

When your threshold has been met, then symptoms begin to appear. It is these symptoms, as I've said before, that we categorize as diseases. But really, they are just names for a collection of what ails us. And of course, if we're always just medicating away the symptoms, how do we know if we're truly getting better?

NEVER MASK THE SYMPTOMS

In my practice, I suggest never masking the symptoms with drugs. Symptoms are our gauge for whether someone is getting well or not.

As I write this, I remember just earlier today when I saw a 5-year-old girl in my practice with head to toe psoriasis. She was itchy, uncomfortable, had bleeding scabs, and couldn't sleep.

The easy choice would have been to recommend she look to her PCP to prescribe cortisone based creams to provide temporary relief and mask the symptoms, but that is not what they came to me for. They had heard I helped many others with her same condition and knew there would be a period of time of having to force the toxins out of her body and not suppress them any longer.

This mother knew that she must heal her daughter's gut and remove food sensitivities from her diet. They understood that the path to wellness would not be as simple as taking a pill and pretending everything was okay on the inside. Instead, they chose to look at the big picture and long-term results…

The story I just shared is an example of one more form of stress on the body that fills up an adult's or child's rain barrel. Please keep in mind that most of us only think about stress from an emotion-based standpoint. We correlate our work, family, and relationships with the level of stress we feel.

However, there are 2 other major stressors on your body that many people don't even think about. We're also never taught them in school, so we pay very little attention to this fact.

DIGESTIVE STRESS

One of those major stresses is your digestive system, or gut. Your gut refers to your stomach, small intestine, large intestine (colon), gut bacteria (microbiome), and overall digestion.

So, if you have any type of candida, bacteria, parasite, or malabsorption issues in your gut, it's going to add to your total stress load.

When your gut is inflamed from any of the reasons I mentioned above, or you're eating foods that you're sensitive to, it can cause an immune reaction. This means your natural defense system begins to attack the food particles inside your intestines causing inflammation and potential damage to your intestinal lining itself (especially in cases such as celiac disease).

Plus, this inflammation in the gut sends signals through your vagus nerve to your brain that something is wrong down there. Your brain then sends you back signals that are interpreted as increased anxiety, nervousness, depression, fatigue, brain fog, or some other byproduct of a deeper underlying imbalance.

The entire body is connected and the sooner we learn this as a society, the better off we will all be.

LEAKY GUT

"Leaky gut" is the cute catch phrase for increased intestinal permeability. This health condition has actually been around since the beginning of time, but conventional medicine only started accepting it over the past decade, so it's only becoming more well known now.

Leaky gut issues are now pervasive in our modern culture since most people have used at least one of the following during their life: Antibiotics, NSAIDs (like Advil), alcohol, birth control pills, and processed food.

The other interesting concept I'm seeing in my practice is that some people never seem to develop a fully balanced microbiome. This means that they may not have been born via a vaginal birth to populate their gut with the proper bacteria, or they may have inherited an imbalanced microbiota from their mother.

Plus, in the first two years of life the intestinal gaps are purposely left wider by nature to allow for immune cells and other beneficial nutrients to pass from the breast milk of the mother to the nursing child and in some cases, these increased intestinal gaps never seem to fully close.

These widened gaps, whether from birth or caused by our environment, can then allow bacteria, yeast, proteins and other pathogens to "leak" directly into your blood stream. This then creates a cascade of events that further heighten your immune system and cause your liver and kidneys to work harder to detoxify.

In my clinical practice, this is one of the main reasons why some people have such a difficult time emptying their rain barrel and decreasing the total stress on their body. Leaky gut is now directly correlated with over 90% of all auto-immune diseases (and I would include almost all dis-eases in general).

Currently, the best and easiest way to test for gut based issues and how well your body is detoxifying is through the Organic Acids Test. For more information about how you can complete this test right at home, please see StephenCabral.com/rbe for a list of up to date lab tests.

VIRUSES & CHRONIC HEALTH CONDITIONS

Another major stressor that fills up your rain barrel is recurrent viruses, bacterial infections, or toxic overload. I'll save the toxic overload issues for the next chapter, but for now let's talk about how viruses and bacteria may be a hidden cause of your current health condition.

Viruses, such as Epstein Barr virus or any of the Herpes based viruses (as well as others), can lay dormant in the body and become reactivated at any time. When this happens your immune system becomes active and imbalanced. Although it's beyond the scope of this book, when you have an imbalance between the Th1 and Th2 branches of your immunes system you begin to suffer from very predictable health struggles.

EXAMPLES OF TH1 IMMUNE SYSTEM DOMINANCE

- Celiac
- Crohn's
- IBS

- Inflammation
- Brain Fog
- Fatigue
- Hashimoto's Thyroiditis
- Rheumatoid Arthritis
- Lichen Planus
- Psoriasis
- Rosacea
- Type 1 Diabetes
- PCOS
- Alzheimer's
- Lupus
- Multiple Sclerosis
- Guillain-Barre Syndrome

EXAMPLES OF TH2 IMMUNE SYSTEM DOMINANCE

- Allergies
- Asthma
- Nasal Drip
- Mucous production
- Atopic Eczema
- Post Nasal Drip
- Hay Fever
- Mastocytosis (histamine intolerance/overload)
- Hives
- Chronic Fatigue Syndrome
- Multiple Chemical Sensitivity
- Autism
- Graves
- Ulcerative Colitis
- Uveitis

The good news is that you don't need to specifically check for immune imbalances or run an intricate cytokine blood work panel at your doctor's office to start. There can be a simpler way to approach the issue.

By following the instructions in this book, you too will have all you need to get started on your healing path. Hopefully, this will save you thousands of dollars and years of struggle getting well.

HOW STRESS AFFECTS US

Now that you know a few of the stressors (work/life/family, gut health, viruses/chronic conditions), let's review how stress actually affects you. This will allow you to reverse engineer the process to finally lift that weight off your shoulders, get healthy and feel free again!

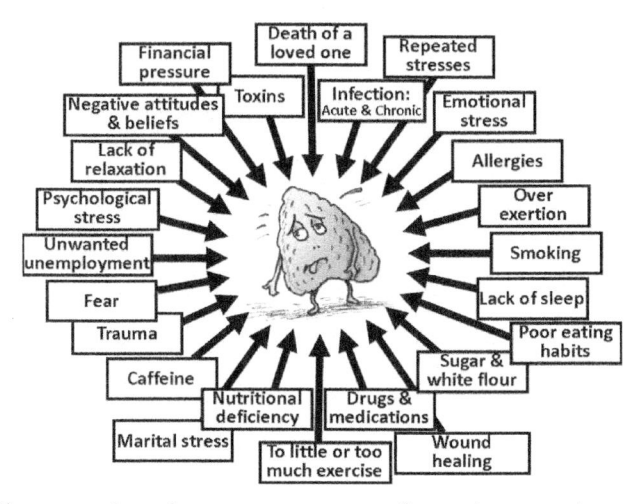

(The image above depicts various sources of stress that wear down your body and weaken your adrenals. Photo Credit: Dr. Lawrence Wilson)

Every system in your body works like a see-saw or teeter totter. What I mean by this is that there are 2 sides to each system of the body and without us knowing it, our body and brain are trying to keep that see-saw balanced at all times.

One example of this when it comes to stress is something called the autonomic nervous system and it's 2 branches: the sympathetic nervous system and the parasympathetic nervous system.

THE SYMPATHETIC NERVOUS SYSTEM (SNS)

The SNS is also referred to as the fight or flight side of your nervous system. When you are stressed it gets turned on and the parasympathetic nervous system (PNS) quiets down. This allows your body to focus on the stress. While this is a good thing and very protective in the short-term, over time it can have serious health repercussions such as:

- Lower metabolism
- Weight gain
- Weakened or imbalanced immunity
- Increased cortisol
- Lowered DHEA, testosterone, progesterone
- Estrogen dominance in women
- Short-term memory loss
- Poor concentration
- Fatigue
- Poor digestion
- Feelings of overwhelm, anxiety, and irritability
- Muscle loss, or tissue/bone breakdown
- Feeling "burnt out"

The reason for all these symptoms of SNS dominance is that humans are only meant to dip in and out of the fight or flight response for short periods of time. Historically, the original humans were either being chased by a predator, enemy, or maybe were in a time of famine. Either way, the stress would end in a relatively short period of time.

However, we currently live in a 24/7 go-go-go society that has us running from one stress to the next. We literally never slow down, unless we're sleeping in bed, and even then far too many people struggle to fall asleep quickly and get a solid 8 hours of uninterrupted sleep every night.

If this sounds like you, then you are missing the key to rejuvenating your body. In order for you to enjoy the opposite of any of the symptoms listed above, you must move into the PNS and out of the stress response. I know this is easier said than done, but I will be teaching you how in the next few pages as well as in the coming chapters.

THE CORTISOL STEAL

When I was 18 year old and still trying to figure out the root cause of my health issues, I had met an "alternative doctor" that had gotten his degree outside of the United States. Having been educated overseas, he spent a significant amount of time studying the pathophysiology of dis-ease and how it comes about.

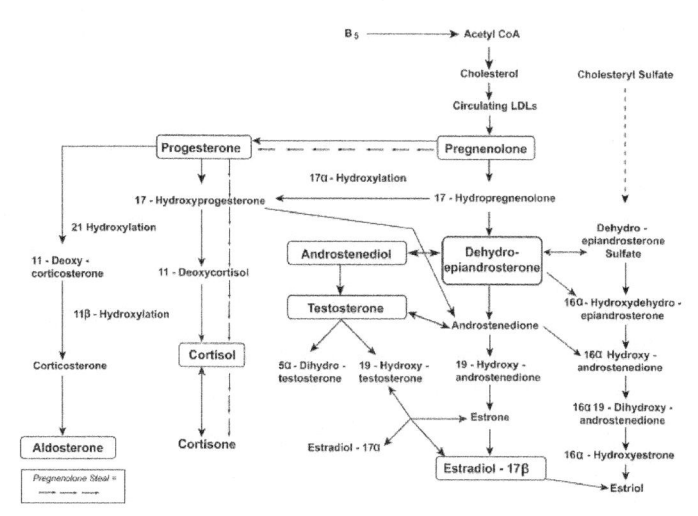

(This exact flow chart above was the visual I needed to finally see how to rebalance you're my body by starting to consciously cut back on stress.)

This doctor showed me the chart above (now used in Functional Medicine), which explains how stress causes massive hormone and immune imbalances, which in turn cause the weight gain and dis-eases we suffer from.

The "cortisol steal" concept explains that when your body is stressed, you automatically begin to preferentially shift available hormone in your body to make more cortisol. The reason for this is cortisol is the hormone that keeps us alive from an evolutionary perspective. Cortisol is responsible for the fight or flight response within the body. It creates a heightened awareness and a constriction of the muscles and blood vessels to prepare us for an attack.

During a much more primitive time in our evolution, this process would keep us safe and allow us to either run from a predator or prepare to attack an oncoming threat. The problem is that in our current culture, the "threat" never ends and we're left with excess adrenaline and cortisol in our blood, as well as the bad mood it creates.

LOWERING OF HORMONES

Another major issue with the cortisol steal is that it can lower your DHEA, testosterone, and progesterone. The reason for this is that when stress is high your nervous system shuttles your hormones into the elevated cortisol (and adrenaline) fight or flight response.

Plus, DHEA and testosterone are anabolic hormones, which work with the parasympathetic nervous system to rejuvenate your body. This predominantly takes place when you're calm and at rest. Unfortunately, there are many men and women out there looking to boost these hormone levels and they're turning to hormone pills, creams, and injections, which are for the most part completely unnecessary.

The reason I don't believe most people need hormone replacement is due to the fact that there's a reason why their hormones dipped in the first place. We now know we can decrease the cortisol steal and allow natural DHEA, progesterone and testosterone to increase on their own. I help men and women every day in my practice combat aging and feelings of fatigue, by helping them to calm the HPA Axis and stress response (we'll cover that in a moment).

THYROID STRESS

There are multiple reasons why you may have a thyroid issue, such as heavy metal toxicity, immune imbalance, food sensitivity reactions, and leaky gut.

However, none of those root causes directly address how the adrenal glands affect the thyroid. After all, it is the adrenal glands that are producing this nor-epinephrine/adrenaline and cortisol.

Although the biochemistry is complicated, the mechanisms by which your thyroid gets weaker from stress are fairly straight forward. When you get into the fight or flight stress response, you begin to produce corticotropic releasing hormone (CRH) and adrenocorticotropic hormone (ACTH) when your brain receives signals of stress. This primes the adrenal actions of producing norepinephrine/adrenaline and cortisol.

HOW YOUR ADRENALS AFFECT YOUR THYROID

(Until conventional medicine re-learns that the adrenals/stress cause the thyroid to malfunction, millions of people will continue to needlessly suffer from thyroid issues.)

The interesting notation here is that when you begin to produce these stress hormones, your thyroid begins to get blocked at the T4 position, as well as causing active T3 thyroid hormone to be converted to the detrimental unusable reverse T3 (rT3) hormone.

The reason why I say this is interesting is because it all makes perfect sense from a holistic health perspective. Your body is not messing up. It is purposely slowing your thyroid in times of stress. This slowing of your thyroid then allows you to conserve calories, gain weight in times of low food supply, and puts you into essentially a protective hibernation state. This very well helped people stay alive longer thousands of years ago.

The problem is that this lowering of our thyroid no longer serves us in the same way, but nonetheless we can't change our natural hormonal processes – we must work in harmony with them.

To do that, we must literally Empty Our Rain Barrel™ of the stresses (life, gut, health conditions) keeping us from living the life we want.

HOW STRESSED ARE YOU?

The most fantastic part of our science today is that we can actually test most of the underlying imbalances leading to dis-ease.

Testing your levels of stress is no different. To find out how stressed you are, we run an at-home saliva lab test that measures cortisol throughout day, along with your DHEA, testosterone, estrogen, and progesterone. It's an amazing lab test that shows you whether your adrenals are suffering and how your endocrine (hormone) system is holding up.

If you believe that both your thyroid and adrenals could be the cause of weight gain, low thyroid, or Hashimoto's, you can a run a combination lab of the same saliva lab test mentioned above, in addition to a blood spot card you can also do right at home. These results will also show you your TSH, T4, T3, and TPO levels.

And finally, if you're looking for a less expensive starter option you can run a Hair Tissue Mineral Analysis, which will show you your levels of autonomic nervous system stress by looking at electrolyte patterns of calcium, magnesium, sodium, and potassium. These minerals react predictably based on SNS and PNS function.

You can find out more about these labs and all other book resources at StephenCabral.com/rbe

IT'S TIME TO RELAX

Now that we know a few of the reasons why it's imperative that we learn to decrease stress in our life, let's talk about some realistic ways to begin doing that.

I'm convinced that although I was prescribed over 3,000 antibiotics before the age of 18, which completely ruined my gut health and immunity, one of the major reasons I got so sick was due to stress. I was simply too hard on myself – about everything.

I was a perfectionist. I wanted to excel at school, sports, and anything I participated in. While it allowed me to do well, I never learned to control it. It wasn't until I realized that I was more stressed than I thought, that I could actually begin the healing process.

After going through my own health struggles, as well as helping thousands of others, I've found these "Stress protocols" to be an essential part of de-stressing. They will not only aid you in recovering faster from any health condition, but they will also clear your mind and make you a happier person!

EXERCISE

I mentioned in the last chapter all the benefits of exercise and how it can help you to alleviate depression, anxiety, panic attacks and other mood disorders, so I won't repeat that here. What I *will say* is that completing even just 10-20 minutes of exercise each day can make a huge difference in reducing stress and resetting your HPA Axis.

MARTIAL ARTS

Kickboxing and martial arts are one of my favorite personal outlets. It's exercise, but it's also a primal way of getting out aggression by kicking and punching. Both men and women in my practice end up loving kickboxing classes and find it to be a therapeutic outlet.

To get started, simply look for an informal kickboxing class at your local gym, hire a boxing/kickboxing instructor, or join a local martial arts dojo of your liking.

WALKING

No one is a bigger proponent of walking than I am… My private wellness clients often joke with me that they feel like a 90-year old patient when I recommend walking as part of their *Personalized Wellness Plan*.

The reason I recommend it is because walking outside, breathing in your environment, and swinging your arms, allows you to shift into that calming parasympathetic nervous system state.

Every single day (unless it's literally raining sideways) I take a break at lunch to walk for 30-60 minutes. It allows me to shift gears, get out of the office, and focus on calming down my body and mind.

SCREAM THERAPY

This type of therapy really does work well for specific people. If you are someone that has a hard time speaking up, expressing your feelings, or you feel like people take advantage of your kind nature, this may be helpful.

It's also being used in more formal psychotherapy to help relieve the wounds of older traumas and repressed memories/emotions. You can seek out a therapist, read more about this topic, or simply begin by screaming into a pillow or when you're alone in your car. It works exceptionally well when you're feeling frustrated and need a healthy outlet. You *do not* want to keep stress bottled up inside.

LAUGHING

Somewhat the opposite of scream therapy, laughing is purposely seeking out situations, friends, and events that make you laugh out loud.

I enjoy listening to certain comedians or old movies I know make me laugh. I also enjoy the time I spend with my long-time friends where we just sit back and joke around light-heartedly.

Laughing is honestly one of the secrets to rebalancing your nervous system, hormones, immunity, and longevity. Make sure you find at least a few times a day where you can enjoy a good laugh!

5-MINUTE MEDITATION

I'll be talking about meditation more in a coming chapter, but we have all noticed that meditation is becoming more and more popular and mainstream. The reason for this is simple – it works!

It's been scientifically verified to reprogram your brain waves in order to switch you out of a high beta-wave state and into a low-beta or theta state. This calms your thought process and allows your body to heal at a deep level.

For beginners, I recommend starting with a basic 5-minute meditation where you just find a comfortable, quiet place to sit and start to focus on your breathing. Simply breathe in through your nose and let it fill up the lower lobes of your lungs which will cause your belly to rise. After that, slowly breathe out through your mouth releasing all the toxins and toxic thoughts. Keep your thoughts for now focused on each slow breath coming in and each slow breath going out.

BETA & THETA WAVE MUSIC

One of my favorite way to switch into a deepened relaxation state is to use Beta and Theta wave sound tracks. These are usually nature based sounds with what's called binaural beats as undertones. This allows for a change in your stress-state brain waves to switch to a calmer low-beta or theta wave state.

Scientific studies have shown that the same brain waves achieved by a longtime Tibetan Monk while meditating can be had by those using these special sound tracks. I also enjoy using them while going for walks. They allow me to get into a state I refer to as, "Waking Meditation." I'm breathing, relaxed, and calm. I'm not focused on anything in particular and I'm just at rest in mind and body.

DANCE TO MUSIC

If you're someone that loves music and dancing then this can be an amazing way to Empty Your Rain Barrel™ of stress. My recommendation is that you listen to upbeat, happy music with lyrics that do not focus on depressing or negative thoughts.

Once you've selected some of your favorite songs, simply close your door, crank up the music, smile, laugh and dance like nobody is watching – remember, you need an outlet to get that stress out!

GENTLE MASSAGE

Most people opt for deep tissue massage, but in order for you to enjoy the relaxation benefits it's crucial you choose medium or lighter pressure. Many people think it's a complete waste of money not to have their massage therapist crank on their body to the point of pain, but that's simply not true.

A deep tissue massage can be beneficial for opening up muscle adhesions and fascia, but it's also highly stimulating to an already stressed nervous system. This is why I opt for lighter pressure and more of a calming massage. It's exactly what stressed people need to unwind, relax, and calm their body and mind.

Adding cranial sacral massage or foot reflexology can also be amazingly effective if you've never experienced them before. I highly recommend making massage (or self-massage) a part of your healthy lifestyle.

THE SOFT ARTS

Combative martial arts and intense training were always referred to as the "hard arts." Practitioners knew they must balance these "hard arts" with the "soft arts" which include yoga, Tai Chi, Qi Gong, and other calming "internal" practices.

For our adrenaline-loving society, we often consider gentle yoga and other soft forms of movement a waste of time. However, nothing could be further from the truth. Ancient wisdom is now backed up by modern science proving that if you go hard all the time, then your body is most likely going to burn out faster.

This means that if you want to live longer, stay healthier, and enjoy a great quality of life, then you must balance high stress living and activities with periods of calming practice.

FLOAT THERAPY

Float therapy is all about relaxation through meditation and floating in isolation tanks. The way these work is through removing external stimulus (light and sound) and allowing some sensory deprivation to help the mind and body to achieve a state of pure relaxation with no distractions. Salts are used in these tanks to help the body float in a very shallow amount of water and achieve a sense of weightlessness, as well as aid in the purification process.

Inside these private tanks, you get to enjoy 60-90 minutes of complete peace and quiet, with no lights, sounds, or distractions.

Float therapy has actually been around since the 1950s and it can be an amazing experience that has left many users reporting an overall greater sense of well-being and less anxiety, depression, fibromyalgia, and stress.

"Floating centers" are becoming more popular and you'll be able to find them in most metropolitan cities. There are also plenty of websites that will teach you how to make you own float tank for home use if that is something you're interested in.

SUPPLEMENTS

We'll be delving deep into nutritional supplements and their healing power in the coming chapters, but for now I wanted to provide you with certain vitamins, minerals, and herbs that have scientific research validating their ability to help you combat stress.

B-Vitamins

The b-vitamin family is particularly helpful when trying to deal with stress. Like the other supplements listed below (minus the adaptogens) all of these nutrients get depleted during times of stress… so obviously, it only makes sense to supplement with what your body is asking for the most.

B-vitamins help improve energy, decrease stress, and improve other processes within the body. They also help boost mood and normal detox processes within your genetics. Look for a good quality "methylated" B-complex with about 50mg of each b-vitamin.

Vitamin C

Vitamin C is crucial for adrenal health and energy. It's also needed for tissue repair, immunity and detoxification.

Zinc

Zinc is one of the most anabolic minerals in the body. It is vital for tissue repair, boosting your immune system, hormones, and healing your gut.

Glutamine

l-Glutamine is the most abundant amino acid in the body and is used for detoxification. Additionally, glutamine is essential for rebuilding bodily tissue and combating stress.

Magnesium

Magnesium is the main mineral that calms the central nervous system and greatly reduces stress.

Cal/Mag

Calcium and magnesium supplementation helps relax your muscles, calms your body, and may be a better solution for those that have higher levels of fatigue (versus magnesium alone).

Phosphatidyl Serine

This unique plant based extract can literally help you lower elevated cortisol levels to calm your body down manually. I'll often use this product with those suffering from stress-induced dis-ease states of sleeplessness, high blood pressure, anxiety, and other high adrenal states.

Adaptogens

Adaptogens have been around since humans first existed. They are mainly plants that are harvested for the roots, leaves, fruit, or other properties unique to that species that help to reduce stress and balance hormones.

Adaptogens also helps to combat stress and bring you to a calmer level when you start to produce more stress hormones. Many adpatogens not only calm you down during a state of stress, but also help with the inverse of giving you more energy when you start to "crash."

Some examples of my favorite adaptogens with a long history of research behind them are:

- Ashwagandha
- Rhodiola
- Siberian Ginseng
- Eleuthero
- Maca

For more details on these products and my up-to-date specific, unbiased recommendations go to StephenCabral.com/rbe

SCHEDULED DOWN TIME

I know it sounds strange, but we've been almost brainwashed to believe that if every minute of our day isn't scheduled with an activity, then we're wasting time or worse, we simply don't know what to do with ourselves when things are calm and quiet!

But, for time-crunched people whose entire day is booked from waking until going to bed, it's crucial you create scheduled down times. I started doing this myself when I realized I would work straight through lunch and by the time I looked up it was mid-afternoon and I hadn't taken a break or even eaten anything since breakfast (and I wondered why I was so tired and would get afternoon headaches!).

To combat this, I had to rework a new lifestyle schedule. It's always a work in progress based on where I'm at in life and how I'm feeling, but now I stop work around 11:30am for a 60-90-minute lunch break.

By that point I've already worked 4 hours and it's time to switch gears. During this time, I'll take my lunch-time walk, do a yoga class, eat lunch outside (weather permitting), read a book, listen to a podcast, or anything that helps me to unwind.

I'll then work for another 3-4 hours before doing my workout for the day and unwinding for another 60-minutes. After my workout in the later afternoon, I'll finish up with my end of the day projects before heading home and truly shutting things down for the night.

Many people seem to do well using a pattern of 50-minutes on, 10-minutes off, and repeat during the work day, but that doesn't work for me. I'm in appointments much of the day, or I'm creating content in the form of podcasts, videos, articles, and books.

All of this is better suited for about 3-hour blocks of time to go deep into that work. If this is the case for you as well, I've found that longer work periods followed by longer breaks to be much more effective than trying to constantly switch between work and rest mode.

The bottom line is that you simply can't work straight through your day without a few scheduled down times that your body can rely on.

Remember, your nervous system works best with rhythms and clear delineations of what "mode" you're in at that moment. So, if you can keep your planned down time and work times within about 30-minutes of the same time each day you will have more energy, better digestion, and a healthier happier mindset!

WEEKEND RECHARGE

It's so important that you take 1-2 days per week to just unplug. This means minimal input – less of everything in terms of technology, email, events, running around, etc.

Whether it's the weekend or just a day or two you're able to get away from major family and work commitments, it's essential you allow your brain and body to rest.

We turn off our cars, computers, TVs, phones, and every other machine we own, but very few of us ever give our mind and body a full day to recharge without expending more "battery life."

If possible, try to pick one day where you're just relaxing and lounging around as much as possible. For bonus credits, try to only check your phone 3x the whole day.

In my house, we use Sundays as a family day to make a fun breakfast at home, take our girls to the park, and just get outside as much as possible.

ARE YOU LESS STRESSED?

The tricky thing about stress is that many of us never know if we're really even that stressed or not... The problem is that we've been stressed for so long, we don't remember what it feels like to not to be stressed!

Luckily, there is a simple device you can purchase that will help you figure out how stressed your body really is. It's called a heart rate variability (HRV) monitor. You may have heard about this type of science before since it's used in common medical devices like ECGs and blood pressure monitors. It works by measuring the variation and length between heartbeats.

For example, when you are stressed, the HRV monitor will result in low frequency (LF) variability between 0.04 to 0.15 Hz. This range has been associated with greater risk for cardiovascular disease, diabetic neuropathy, SIDS, and a host of other health conditions associated with greater sympathetic nervous system dominance.

Conversely, when you're in a HRV measured state of high frequency (HF) activity (0.15 to 0.40 Hz) it shows more of a parasympathetic nervous system dominance, which is associated with a relaxed state. This means your body is more at ease and less stressed.

In an ideal world, you should aim to be in this state as much as possible. The two most important times to be in the high frequency state is while eating and before bed. This assures that you will digest and absorb your food better, as well as fall into a deep restorative sleep.

I provide my HRV monitor recommendations on this book's corresponding resource web page. If you're trying to optimize your health and you're looking to see how stressed your body is throughout the day, this device may be worth considering.

It's also going to give you the data you need to see how quickly you're recovering from any stress-based dis-ease, as well as how much of an effect any of the treatments above are having on your levels of stress.

CLOSING THE LOOP ON STRESS

None of the suggestions mentioned above are meant to be quick fixes.

I simply want to get you thinking about how you can be more well-rounded and get more out of life, because when you're enjoying life and doing things that you feel are fun, stress disappears!

The mind is a very powerful entity and it's your job to check in with it more about how you're feeling, what your levels of stress are, and how you can avoid the "triggers" that cause you the most tension. When you begin to become more aware, you've found one of the most profound factors in transforming your life…

Go easy on yourself, this is a journey of self-exploration and discovery that is never ending – Enjoy the process!

For all lab choices, supplement recommendations, product reviews and other recommendations made in this book go to: StephenCabral/rbe

EMPTY YOUR RAIN BARREL™ STRESS ACTION PLAN

The best way to truly reduce stress is by going after the underlying root causes of the stress. This means assessing whether your stress is from work/life emotions, digestive system issues, or from a history of viruses and chronic illness. (It is possible that all 3 will need to be addressed.)

Once you've done an honest assessment, it's now time to pick 1 of these 3 levels to begin to Empty Your Rain Barrel™ of stress:

1. CHOOSE A LAB TO FIND THE ROOT CAUSE

You can decide to get direct data on what exactly is off in your body and then go about correcting these issues. You may choose to work with a local Functional Medicine doctor or practitioner, or with our online practice to complete these lab tests.

2. COMPLETE A 21-DAY DETOX

By completing 21 days of an elimination diet and using the specific supplements your body needs to function at a higher level, you'll be able to better assess how much more work you'll need to get well, lose the weight, or simply feel alive again!

Often, this 21-day detox and the maintenance plan is all people need to completely rebalance their body. You can choose any Functional Medicine detox you feel is the best fit for you, or you can go to DrCabralDetox.com for details on what I use in my practice.

3. CHOOSE 1 DE-STRESSING TECHNIQUE

Choose any one of the calming practices from this chapter and commit to it for just 21 days. This will allow you to begin to make that one relaxation based technique a permanent part of your life. You can always add on other relaxation techniques after mastering that first one!

Toxins: Part 1
How to Remove, Reduce, and Eliminate Environmental Toxins in Your Life

One of the scariest things has to be when you finally figure out you've been lied to for most of your life..

You grow up thinking that the government, corporations, teachers, doctors, and many other organizations like this have your best interest at heart.

The truth is that this is simply *not the case*.

Teachers and doctors for the most part try to do their best to help educate you, but they've been misled themselves by private interest groups like big corporations that only care about one thing – Money.

So we haven't been told some of the big, important truths, especially about the state of our world. When you finally come to accept this as the truth, you can begin to see what a toxic world we live in and how we got here. The next step is realizing you most likely have 212 or more cancer- causing toxins floating around or stored in the tissues of your body.[1]

Many of these come from personal products, pesticides, eating toxin containing foods, drinking or washing food in toxic water, breathing pollution, car exhaust – All of these things and more.

For example, of the chemicals found in personal care products the data has shown:

- 884 are toxic
- 146 cause tumors
- 218 cause reproductive complications
- 314 cause biological mutation
- 376 cause skin and eye irritations[2]

This is no longer speculation. It's fact, and it gets even scarier. Did you know that over 90% of America's water systems contain cancer-causing chemicals as well.[3,4]

If you want to read all kinds of fascinating facts on toxins in the average home, personal products, and much more, I love the website called Environmental Alternatives. Check out their blog called "Facts and Statistics on Toxins."[5]

Just like the *National Geographic* article I shared earlier, no one wants to believe they're slowly being poisoned, but we are..

The National Geographic article is just one of thousands highlighting the dangerous world we live in. The problem is that since we can't see the majority of these toxins with our own two eyes, it makes staying clear of them that much more difficult.

(Note: This information is not meant to scare, but rather light a fire under you to get moving, get healthy, and make sure you share this message with others!)

To make your job easier, I'll be listing the major home, office, and environmental toxins to watch out for and their alternatives in a moment.

I'm also going to try to do it in as simple a manner as possible. This chapter literally started out as over 100 pages itself, but the finished version you see now is about 1/3rd of that – while still relating the most important chemicals for you to know about to keep you and your family healthy.

So, instead of telling you what every harmful ingredient does to your body, I just list what to stay away from and which ones are best. This will then allow you to dig deeper into the research on each toxin if you choose to later.

I also broke this chapter up into 2 parts. The 1st part explains what toxins to stay away from and the healthy alternatives for products you use every day such as toothpastes, shampoos, moisturizers, etc. The 2nd part explains how to begin removing some of those already accumulated toxins from your body!

First, I want to explain why it's absolutely imperative that you avoid these chemicals at all costs and do your best to systematically empty them from your blood, body, and brain.

I know I mentioned previously the effects of plastics, pesticides, heavy metals and other toxins in the environment on your health, but I'd like to help you better understand that now.

When a man-made toxin enters your body, it acts like a foreign invader causing a war-like environment inside you. It can assault and damage your intestines, liver, organs, joints, or get lodged in your brain. When this happens, an immune response is mounted and inflammation sets in. And as I said earlier, deadly dis-eases of all kinds begin with inflammation.

This process will look like the symptoms of a disease that you've been diagnosed with. Or worse, doctors can't find out what is wrong with you because your bloodwork looks fine. I've been there, and I know how frustrating that can be…

That's why it's essential that you take back control of your own body and begin to Empty Your Rain Barrel™. It's the simplest and fastest way to get back on track. You may need to do more detoxification in the future, but there is no better place to start since this detoxification work must be done no matter what.

The great news is that we know what we have to do. 6,000 years ago Ayurvedic Medicine taught us the foundation of detoxification through their Pancha Karma therapies. Today, we can combine that with Functional Medicine lab testing and nutritional supplements to give your body the raw material it needs to fight back.

Remember, as explained earlier, with 77,000+ man-made chemicals permeating the environment every day, and more coming all the time, stopping them is not a possibility. What we *can do* is remove them from the body.

So, our job is to first empty our rain barrels and then keep our levels low by quarterly 7-21 day detoxes and following the DESTRESS™ Protocol on a daily basis as best as we can. This is how we keep dis-ease and weight gain away.

And now that you're learning how to Empty Your Rain Barrel™ with the previous portions of the DESTRESS™ Protocol, it's time to show you what items to avoid when trying to lower your toxic load in the future. After that, I'll teach you simple methods to begin safely drawing out the toxins you have internally, using all natural treatments you can do right at home or at a local wellness center.

AVOID THESE TOXIC PRODUCTS TO LOWER YOUR BURDEN

As you read the list of common products below, please do not get overwhelmed. The first reaction will always be to feel it's all too much to handle. However, my advice is to simply relax into the process and understand that deep healing is a journey.

If you're feeling anxious, choose just one at a time to begin to substitute for a healthier option. Within a few months you'll be pleasantly surprised at how much you've accomplished!

SHAMPOO, SOAPS & CONDITIONERS

Believe it or not, the chemicals that make your bath products foam up and create "suds" are actually known cancer-causing substances like Triclosan and Diethanolamine (DEA). There are many others (listed below) that have also been linked to cancer, hormone disruption, and other health issues. My highest recommendation is to read your labels and stay clear of these ingredients.

TOXIC BATH INGREDIENTS

- Sodium Laurel Sulfate
- Fermaldehyde
- Triclosan
- Dioxane
- Diethanolamine
- Phalthates
- PCBS
- Parabens
- PEG-6

BEST SHAMPOO, SOAP & CONDITIONER ALTERNATIVES

One important fact that is often overlooked is that you really shouldn't be washing your hair and scalp on a daily basis. It dries it out and can damage your hair. Try to cut back to every other day or just 1-2 times a week as able. This will ensure that no matter what product you're using it's not building up in your system.

In terms of natural alternative products, I recommend these brands for shampoos and conditioners:

- Soap for Goodness Sake
- Makes 3 Organics
- Opas
- Himalaya
- Dr. Bronner
- Attitude
- Avalon Organics
- Baby Mantra
- Baja Baby

There are many others, but these (currently) meet the criteria for toxic free products you can trust.

Please keep in mind that as you're reading through this chapter every product I recommend will be listed and up-to-date on the resource page: StephenCabral.com/rbe

For soaps, I prefer people to switch over to natural face scrubs if they currently have acne or oil build up, and then soaps that contain coconut, olive oil, or shea butter for daily use. Many people also enjoy the ancient technique of using oil to cleanse their face while hydrating it at the same time.

For soaps, I recommend the same brands as I did above for shampoos and conditioners.

MAKE UP

The average woman is walking around right now wearing an estimated 63 disease causing chemicals on her skin.

Make-up has become so toxic that the US Researchers Report stated 1 in 8 ingredients (out of 82,000) contained known cancer or hormone disrupting chemicals. This is the dirty industry secret that cosmetic companies don't want you to know about.

The issue with make-up is that your skin is porous. This allows any creams, lotions, hormones, chemicals, or anything else placed on it to move directly through the skin and into the bloodstream. Shockingly, this is actually worse than swallowing some toxins, since during digestion your liver will typically be able to filter some of the chemicals before they fully circulate into your blood stream.

This is *not the case* when applying products directly on your skin. The best rule of thumb is to make sure that *if it is not food grade and you can't eat it, then do not put it on your skin.*

As a side note, your skin actually works so well as a transportation vehicle into your blood that all ancient forms of medicine actually used to infuse herbs into oils and then apply them directly to the skin. These healers knew that a few teaspoons of that oil would be adsorbed and would help those with weak digestive systems that couldn't swallow or tolerate ingesting herbs internally.

Here are a list of chemicals to watch out for in your make-up (many are similar to the bath products):

TOXIC MAKE-UP INGREDIENTS

- BHA and BHT
- Coal tar dyes: p-phenylenediamine and colours (listed as "CI" followed by a five digit number)
- DEA-related ingredients
- Dibutyl phthalate
- Formaldehyde-releasing preservatives
- Parabens

- Parfume (a.k.a. "fragrance")
- PEG compounds
- Petrolatum
- Siloxanes
- Sodium laureth sulfate
- Triclosan

(This source list was provided by http://davidsuzuki.org/issues/health/science/toxics/dirty-dozen-cosmetic-chemicals/)

BEST MAKE-UP ALTERNATIVE

- Maia's
- Mineral Fusion
- Beauty Counter
- Rejuva Minerals
- W3LL

(Note: To see how your current make-up or cosmetics stack up you can search their toxicity score at http://www.ewg.org/skindeep/)

MOISTURIZERS

Just like make-up, the same dangers apply to moisturizers and lotions due to the porous nature of your skin. However, the other issue with these products is that they can block the respiration of your skin. This actually means your skin can't breathe as well (remember it's a living organ!), which can further contribute to a build-up of toxins in your system.

The reason this build-up can occur is because your skin is the largest excretory organ in your body. Its job is to remove waste. So by using moisturizers that block this natural process, you are harming one of your body's most important detoxification systems.

Please note that there is some crossover on all these lists. You'll see some repeats on all the skin care products. Simply read your ingredient labels to confirm they are free of the toxins listed.

TOXIC MOISTURIZER INGREDIENTS

- Resorcinol
- Hydroquinone
- Petrolatum
- Xylene
- Toluene
- Mineral oil
- Liquid paraffin
- Methylisothiazolinone
- Oxybenzone
- Parabens
- Synthetic colors
- Fragrance
- Phthalates
- Triclosan
- Sodium lauryl sulfate (SLS) / Sodium laureth sulfate (SLES)
- Formaldehyde
- Toluene
- Mercury
- Paraphenylenediamine (PPD)
- Polyethylene glycol (PEG
- Silicone-derived emollients
- Talc

(This source list was provided by http:///.treehugger.com/organic-beauty/20-toxic-ingredients-avoid-when-buying-body-care-products-and-cosmetics.html)

BEST MOISTURIZER ALTERNATIVES

My highest recommendation for moisturizers is to use an organic food based oil. The reason for this recommendation is simple. Oil helps hydrate the skin at a deeper tissue level, whereas most moisturizers merely block your current skin's oils from coming out. Here are a few of my suggestions:

- Argan Oil
- Jojoba oil
- Carrot Seed oil
- Apricot Seed oil
- Sesame oil (body)
- Coconut oil (body)

Some of my favorites for the face are argon oil, apricot seed oil, carrot seed oil, or jojoba oil. Coconut and sesame oil are also great moisturizers for the body and cost a lot less. I would suggest experimenting with a few face (and body) oils to see which ones work best for your skin. Please try to choose organic, cold processed, first pressed and stored in a dark-tinted glass container.

DEODORANT

Just like certain moisturizers, deodorants can block toxins from escaping from your skin. Antiperspirants compound this fact by not allowing you to sweat out the dangerous chemicals your body is trying to expel.

To make matters worse, you have lymph nodes right under the skin of your armpits that work every day to kill toxins and force them out of the body. Blocking this natural process can be quite harmful in the long-run.

Plus, most antiperspirants contain aluminum as the main ingredient to prevent perspiration. And since we know aluminum can cause auto-immune and brain based issues, it is important to avoid applying this toxin on a daily basis.

Other ingredients in deodorant and skin care products also have been linked directly to breast cancer, prostate issues, and pregnancy complications. Now, I do understand that most people don't want to have body odor. So, here are my suggestions…

First, once you begin to Empty Your Rain Barrel™ and detoxify, most people will notice that they no longer have the same level of body odor as before and some even report they have no body odor at all!

Second, there are natural alternatives to harmful deodorants and antiperspirants. I will give you those names and ingredients to look for after we list what to watch out for. My recommendation is to avoid these harmful deodorant ingredients:

- Aluminum
- Parabens
- Steareths
- Triclosan
- Propylene Glycol
- TEA and DEA
- Artificial Colors & Dyes[6]

BEST DEODORANT ALTERNATIVES

The best brands use activated charcoal to absorb moisture, and then use coconut oil and essential oils like lavender to balances your pH and kill the bacteria on the skin which causes odor. My current non-toxic suggestions are:

- Piper Wai
- Truly's

- Bali Secrets
- BeGreen
- Purely Great
- Honestly pHresh

Please keep in mind that the cosmetic and beauty product industry changes fast so there will always be new updates every few months on the products deemed toxin-free at StephenCabral.com/rbe

TOOTHPASTE AND MOUTH WASH

Oral care is another huge area to be wary of. The tiny capillaries in your mouth allow for the direct transport of certain nutrients (and unfortunately chemicals) directly into your blood stream.

Again, this works exceptionally well for sublingual supplements, but is detrimental when your toothpaste, mouth wash, or other oral care product contains cancer causing carcinogens and other chemicals. Just like with the soaps and shampoos, the best thing to do is make sure you don't have any chemicals in there that may act as foaming agents. Here is a list of items to watch out for:

TOXIC TOOTHPASTE & MOUTH WASH INGREDIENTS

- Triclosan
- Sodium Lauryl Sulfate (SLS)
- Artificial Sweeteners
- Fluoride
- Propylene Glycol (mineral oil)
- Diethanolamine (DEA)
- Microbeads (These are plastic beads!)
- Chlorhexidine
- Alcohol
- Hexetidine (oraldene)
- Methyl Salicylate

- Benzalkonium Chloride
- Cetylpyridinium Chloride
- Methylparaben[7]

BEST TOOTHPASTE & MOUTH WASH ALTERNATIVES

For toothpaste alternatives, you can simply make your own using baking soda, hydrogen peroxide (optional for whitening), peppermint oil, and some tea tree oil. You can also add a little stevia if needed for sweetness. For pre-made recipes like this you may purchase brands that are fluoride and chemical-free at your local health conscious grocery food store like Whole Foods or Sprouts.

Here are some of my favorite fluoride-free toothpaste brands, but please see this book's online resource page for up to date recommendations since brands do change all the time:

- Jason
- Dr. Brite
- Redmond
- Dr. Bronner's
- Lucky Teeth organic toothpaste and mouthwash

Also, as a traditional mouth wash alternative, I can't recommend oil pulling enough. You can use either a sesame or coconut oil and simply swish the oil around in your mouth for about 10-minutes every morning when you wake up. Not only will it kill bacteria and unhealthy microbes living there, but it will freshen your breath and whiten your teeth!

Whenever you purchase an oil for pulling (or eating) look for these notations:

- Organic (non-GMO)
- First pressed

- Cold pressed
- Extra virgin (especially olive oil)

LAUNDRY DETERGENT

Did you know most clothes are made with harmful dyes and treated with other chemicals to preserve their color?

The same dyes and chemicals that you would never eat can unfortunately be absorbed through direct contact with your skin the same exact way I explained with skin-care products above.

The good news is that washing new clothes a few times before wearing them will draw out many of those initial cancer-causing chemicals. Whenever possible, try to look for more natural clothing alternatives made out of organic cotton, bamboo, hemp or other safe, sustainable materials. They look the same and feel great on your skin!

Now that you know clothes themselves can actually harbor hidden toxins, here's a list of laundry detergent chemicals to be weary of. The residue from these detergents can remain on your clothing and again be absorbed through your skin.

(As an aside, try to also find a chemical-free dry cleaner if you have your dress clothes dry cleaned and pressed since dry cleaning chemicals are some of the most toxic byproducts for both the environment and your body.)

TOXIC CHEMICALS IN DETERGENT

- Sodium lauryl sulfate (SLS)/sodium laureth sulfate (SLES)
- Sodium dodecyl sulfate
- Sulfuric acid, monododecyl ester, sodium salt
- Sodium salt sulfuric acid

- Monododecyl ester sodium salt sulfuric acid
- A13-00356
- Akyposal SDS
- Aquarex ME
- 1,4-dioxane
- NPE (nonylphenol ethoxylate)
- Phosphates

BEST LAUNDRY DETERGENT ALTERNATIVES

Although not all brands may be perfect, reducing the toxin exposure is a step in the right direction. Here are some of the cleanest detergents available:

- Green Shield
- Earth Friendly
- BioKleen
- Attitude
- Better Life
- Fit Organic
- Green Shield
- 7th Generation
- Sun & Earth

COOKING PRODUCTS

Since I do a lot of Hair Tissue Mineral Analysis (HTMA) testing, I get to look at heavy metal levels for patients on a daily basis. One disturbing trend I see is the increasing amount of aluminum in people's hair samples.

Since we use aluminum-free scissors and we've tested our own double blind samples, I know these results are legitimate. Plus, aluminum toxicity is one of the major health issues being discussed right now. One reason for this is the free radical damage that is caused when mercury, aluminum, lead, or other heavy metals accumulate in your body.

Low levels seem to be fine, but once you exceed your rain barrel tolerance, damage begins to occur and symptoms become evident. With Alzheimer's and dementia on the rise and the toxicity link to those brain-based issues, it makes a lot of sense to get tested and ensure you're removing as much aluminum from your life as possible.

Since cooking pans, spatulas, and aluminum foil are mainstays of most households, it's important to look at these items first. When you cook in aluminum coated pans and scrape the pan you're releasing these heavy metals directly into your food. The same holds true for cooking or wrapping your heated food in aluminum foil.

BEST ALUMINUM COOKING ALTERNATIVES

- Copper pans
- Cast Iron
- Ceramic
- Glass

PLASTIC WRAPS

I know that we're all busy. I also understand that you most likely don't have a lot of time to cook – I don't either. But, I must warn you that using a microwave and heating your food that's been covered with plastic wrap releases PCBs, PVC, polyethylene, polypropylene, and other known cancer-causing agents directly into your food.

Plus, all of those "microwave safe bags" are *not safe*. You're literally microwaving plastic chemicals into your food. When food marketing companies say they're microwave safe, they only mean that the bag will not melt in the microwave – It doesn't mean they are safe for you… just the microwave!

Those plastic bags are also marketed to be dropped into boiling water at high temperatures, which still releases the same toxins as plastic wrap into your food. You then consume the food, unknowingly eating cancerous chemicals. With this type of deceptive marketing, is it any wonder why cancer rates are spiking every decade?

BEST PLASTIC WRAP ALTERNATIVES

- Don't use a microwave
- Reheat in an oven or toaster oven
- Heat in the morning and place in a heat-safe container that keeps your food warm
- For leftovers, use a glass jar and safe cover (or wait before cooling to use a plastic cover and do not let it touch the hot food)

BABY & CHILDREN PRODUCTS

Having two young girls, I know first-hand what it's like trying to keep everything they pick up out of their mouths. They seem to want to taste every object they touch…

Because of this, it's very important to choose children's products that are non-toxic and safe for them to play with. You may not know this, but products made overseas can contain lead, harmful paints, and heavy metals which can flake off or come off in your child's mouth.

Additionally, many fabrics, dolls, and toys come with flame retardant chemical solutions that are known cancer causing carcinogens. This is actually much worse for young children, since their immune systems are not fully developed and due to their overall size, they cannot combat the large amount of toxins in our environment.

It's also why we're seeing such a large increase in childhood diseases. Plus, some materials are so toxic it has even caused death in rare cases.[8]

Instead of listing all the toxins, I'd rather point you to one website that has done all the work for you. Remember, since toys and other non-edible products are not meant for human consumption a full list of ingredients in each object is not required to be given. Here are the most toxic toys to watch for:

MOST TOXIC TOYS

- Plastic dolls
- Plastic toy parts that are easy to break off
- Painted toys that can chip or be swallowed
- Toys with fragrances
- Clays and paints with synthetic dyes
- Flame retardant coated toys or fabrics

BEST CHILDREN'S TOY ALTERNATIVES

- Wooden toys
- Non-painted, or food safe
- Organic, food based clays
- Non-toxic markers and paints

BEST WEBSITES FOR ADDITIONAL INFORMATION

- Healthy Child Healthy World (healthychild.org)
- Healthy Stuff (www.ecocenter.org/healthy-stuff/)
- U.S. Public Interest Research Group (uspirg.org/news/usf/trouble-toyland)
- Consumer Product Safety Commission (cpsc.gov/Newsroom/News-Releases/)

Although it's difficult to be perfect, by simply being more aware of what toys your child is playing with, you'll be cutting down on their total toxic load and also be limiting their exposure to potentially harmful manufacturing practices.

TAP WATER

Wouldn't it be great to drink fresh water that came right out of your tap?

It would, but that day is still not here...

Don't get me wrong, I'm grateful that our water is typically free from parasites, bacteria, and for the most part drinkable, but it still falls short of being healthy for you.

A recent investigation by the *Associated Press* showed that every municipal city water that was tested came back positive for pharmaceutical drugs. I bet you didn't expect to hear that? The reason for this pollution of our water with drugs like antidepressants is due to the fact that people often flush their prescriptions. Also, when you urinate much of the active and inactivated forms of the drug also comes out in your urine.

You may still be asking yourself how do the drugs in your toilet water end up in your tap water. It's a great question and one we've been deceived about for a long time. You see, your drinking water often comes from sewage waste. You heard that correctly. Sewage water is collected, filtered, "decontaminated" and then recirculated back into the drinking water through your kitchen and bathroom faucets. This is actually so common worldwide that *CNN News* way back in 2014 did a piece called, "*From Toilet to Tap: Drinking Recycled Waste Water.*"

It's no longer a reality that all of our water comes from these beautiful reservoirs of pristine water. And even if they do, your city adds chlorine to kill bacteria. Again, this is extremely helpful to keep you from drinking harmful pathogens, but the same chlorine that kills bacteria in the water also kills healthy beneficial bacteria (probiotics) in your gut.

Hopefully, it's now starting to make sense as to why so many people have gut dysfunction and poor bacterial balance. When you couple this with the fact that 80% of your immune system lies in and outside of your intestines and effects every disease known to man, you can begin to understand how everything we come in contact with can either build us up or break us down.

Besides chlorine, fluoride is typically added to tap water. Some people will make the argument that fluoride is essential for healthy teeth. I'm not one of those people, and the research just isn't there. Humans (and animals) have always lived without the consumption of added synthetic fluoride and maintained strong and healthy teeth throughout their lives.

Dr. Weston A. Price and others have shown that it is the addition of processed foods, poor oral hygiene, and toxicity based health issues that causes poor dental health.[9]

Regardless of which side of the argument you stand by, the fact is that fluoride should not be swallowed. So, even if you believe it's necessary for your teeth, you still wouldn't eat or drink it. It's a known poison that can kill you (or cause serious harm) in a pea-sized quantity. This is why there's a warning on all fluoridated tubes of toothpastes.

Additionally, fluoride has been known for decades to lower thyroid gland function. It's even been used to treat Graves' disease (overactive thyroid function) in some European countries, since it's been studied and shown to effectively weaken thyroid output.

In addition to fluoride, some water systems are being filtered by using aluminum. Aluminum acts like a surfactant which grabs on to other heavy metals (such as lead) and pulls them down to the bottom of the tank. What's left is water with less heavy metals in it – Except aluminum, which is often higher than before the water was treated.

Although there's much more to cover when it comes to tap water (like pesticide runoff, etc.), the bottom line is that it's not clean, nor pure. Because of this I recommend looking into a good quality water filter or source for natural spring water.

Also, remember that most bottled water companies deceitfully use straight tap water that has been minimally filtered, You can do better filtration at home for a lot less money. Below is a list of effective water filtration systems in order of most expensive to least expensive.

BEST WATER ALTERNATIVES

- Multi-step water filtration system
  (This is typically a 5-step or more system of purifying all contaminants in your water.)
- Reverse osmosis under the counter filtration system
  (I recommend this over distillation, since less water is used and it's a far easier alternative.)
- Berkey countertop filter
- Zero or Therasage water pitchers

Another nice option is looking into a whole house water filtration system. These systems can be pricy, but they represent a one-time cost. They also allow all the incoming water to your home to be filtered before it comes out of your kitchen faucet, shower or bath. This then saves you from having to purchase other filters for your bath and shower as well. If you know you'll be living in the same home for the next 5+ years it may be worth the investment.

To listen to my full podcast detailing water filter recommendations, go to StephenCabral.com/rbe

SHOWER & BATH FILTERS

Now that you know how toxic your tap water really is, I want to provide you with one more note.

I mentioned earlier that the water coming out of your pipes contains chlorine. This becomes a major problem when you shower or bathe. Besides being drying and harmful to your hair and skin, it actually has a much more problematic effect.

Chlorine comes out of your shower (and hot bath) as a gas. These vapors then remain in the air while you shower and are inhaled. At this point, the chlorine has now become a toxic gas that gets drawn directly into your lungs and passed into your blood stream. The long-term effects of this poison is something that can weaken your liver's detox abilities (reducing glutathione), overall respiratory health, and energy production.

So to combat the chlorinated gas in your shower and bath, I recommend keeping the whole family (including children) safe by installing a showerhead and bath filter. I'm certainly not a skilled tradesman and I was able to do it in less than 1 minute.

BEST SHOWER & BATH FILTERS

- Aquabliss (You keep your current showerhead)
- Sprite (Replaces your existing showerhead)
- Culligan (Small shower head and filter all-in-one)
- CUZn Bath filter (Slides right over the bath spout)

For my Cabral Concept podcast on shower and bath filters, as well as current recommendations go to StephenCabral.com/rbe

I know many of these items seem like a lot to deal with, but as I suggested earlier, simply make small changes one at a time. This allows you to ease into the process. Plus, most of these changes are honestly easy lifestyle switches that you'll never even notice after you make the initial switch.

Once you remove these main toxicities from your life, you can always look at additional alternative healthy lifestyle practices. And, if you're on my email newsletter list or listen in to my podcast, you'll be sure to get all those action tips each and every week.

So now that you know how to cut way back on the amount of health-robbing chemicals coming into your body, it's time to discuss how you can remove the ones that are currently there.

I was fortunate enough to learn these practices, which have been all but lost except for a few Ayurvedic and ancient healing clinics. It was always my goal to be able to share what I learned from spending time overseas learning the best of every form of medicine.

Part 2 details a few easy-to-implement techniques that will greatly reduce your total toxic load and help Empty Your Rain Barrel™!

Toxins: Part 2
How to Remove, Reduce, and Eliminate Environmental Toxins in Your Body

Now that you know many of the common household products to stay away from, let's move on to how you can actually Empty Your Rain Barrel™ and remove some of those toxins currently stuck in your body.

I'll be sharing the specific nutrition and supplementation protocol to bind up those toxins and help your liver neutralize and expel them in the last part of this book, but one thing you have to keep in mind is that by using certain external detoxification protocols, you can actually help the process move along much faster.

The reason for this is your liver, kidneys, skin, and lungs are working as fast and efficiently as they can to dismantle those toxicities on their own, but they could use some help.

Although these natural detox treatments have been used as far back as 6,000 years ago in India, and then in China, Egypt, and Greece, they have largely been forgotten.

MODERN DAY PANCHA KARMA

It was in Sri Lanka that I first discovered Pancha Karma. This discovery would change the way I viewed health and medicine forever. Up until this time, I thought we should always add more (herbs, vitamins, etc.) in order to help someone get well.

As I mentioned earlier, Pancha Karma truly is the closest thing we have to the *Fountain of Youth*. This has been known throughout the ages and my goal with this book is to allow you to enjoy a simplified, less expensive version that you can implement easily on a daily basis and then eventually on a larger scale seasonally.

So, although my internships in the East involved extensive half and full day detox patient protocols that lasted a week or more, what I've come to realize is that you can replicate these great results over time (instead of front loaded) by using the same techniques in just a fraction of the time and cost.

Below, I will list some of those treatments that you can do right at home. Most take less than 5-minutes and cost just $10 - $100.

SELF-MASSAGE

Self-massage, or Abhyanga as referred to in Ayurveda, is a style of massage used to improve circulation and help drain your lymphatic fluid of toxins.

The example I'm about to give you is the same type of massage you'd receive in an authentic Pancha Karma treatment – But you can use this therapy right at home before you get in the shower or before bed.

The idea is to mimic the technique of a manual lymphatic drainage massage. This means you are trying to manually move toxins right out of your body through your lymph, which is the fluid that helps transport waste. Not only is this highly effective, it boosts every health mechanism in your body.

The best way to do this self-massage is by purchasing the same type of oil you'd use in Ayurvedic massage treatments. If you do not know your Dosha type (body's constitution) you do not have to pick a Vata, Pitta, or Kapha specific herbal oil. Instead, you can simply purchase a bottle of organic cold pressed sesame oil.

In the next section under dry brushing I will explain the movement of the self-massage, which can be mimicked with a dry brush as well.

DRY BRUSHING

Dry brushing your skin may sound strange, but just like Ayurvedic self-massage, it is meant to stimulate and move the lymphatic fluid.

In my practice, I recommend that dry brushing be done right before your morning shower. I find this is the best time to wake up the lymph and circulation.

The reason for lymphatic congestion in the first place is that your lymphatic fluid works on a manual pump. This means that unless you are actively moving your lymph, it stays stagnant.

And since most people sit during the day, you can begin to see how waste gets stuck and pools in your body. This is also why I believe you'll be hearing much more about the lymph system in the future as natural health minded practitioners rediscover its importance in maintaining and restoring proper health.

So, if you've never heard of dry brushing before, I'd like to briefly walk you through this practice.

You'll need a pair of silk gloves (raw rough silk) or a dry brush (which is what I typically recommend). Gently press the gloves or brush down on your skin (about 3mm depth) and stroke along your body towards your heart. As long as you always keep the dry brush strokes light and moving in the direction towards the heart, you'll be doing it correctly.

If you want to get more technical for your self-massage or dry brushing, my recommendation is to watch the online video tutorials on the resource page, or follow these directions:

3-MINUTE MORNING DRY BRUSHING DRILL
LOWER BODY

1. Use the dry brush for all strokes against your skin and apply light, even pressure
2. You can use straight strokes towards the heart or circular movements
3. Pick the brush up after the stroke is complete and start again – Do not stroke away from the heart
4. Stroke 3-7 times in one area before moving to the next spot
5. Begin at your knee caps and stroke up towards your groin
6. Continue to move from knee cap to groin all around your thigh until the whole upper leg is finished
7. Repeat on the other thigh and buttocks (towards lower back)
8. Next, stroke from your ankle up to your knee cap just like you did with the upper thigh. Repeat on the other side
9. Now, stroke up from the ankle to your groin in one long even movement over the whole leg. Complete on both sides.

UPPER BODY

1. Use the same technique as the lower body
2. Raise your arm above your heart and stroke from your wrist to your armpit
3. Repeat on the other arm
4. Use the long handle brush to stroke from your lower back and upper shoulders towards your armpit.
5. Gently brush your chest towards your centerline or armpits
6. Use the brush in a clockwise direction on your stomach making 7 circles around your navel (belly button)
7. Place the brush down and use your finger tips with light pressure to stroke down your neck from your jawline to your clavicles (collar bones)

By getting into the habit of using the above technique every morning with either massage oil or a dry brush, I have no doubt you will begin to feel your energy lift from the manual lymph drainage of toxins and the increased oxygenation of your tissues!

EPSOM SALT BATHS

Epsom salt baths are pretty much everyone's favorite.

The reason I say this is because taking an Epsom salt bath is all about relaxation and calming the nerves. It's taking some much deserved quiet time for yourself to unwind and shut off the fight or flight response.

The reason this treatment works so well is because Epsom salt (named after the natural spring in England) is composed of magnesium and sulfate. Magnesium is a renowned mineral with massive amounts of clinical data showing its effectiveness in calming the central nervous system. Taking an Epsom salt bath before bed can also help you relax and sleep easier. The sulfate in this "salt" solution helps to detoxify the body because sulfur is an essential component of Phase 2 liver detoxification.[10]

And since your skin is porous, it allows for the subdermal transfer of the magnesium and sulfur in the water to be absorbed directly into your blood stream. This makes Epsom salt baths a simple, stress-free way to naturally supplement with two necessary ingredients for mental and physical well being!

HOW TO TAKE AN EPSOM SALT BATH

Although you will need a bathtub, taking an Epsom salt bath is completely hands off. Here are the simple instructions for enjoying a little spa relaxation right at home:

1. Turn on the tub with the hottest water you can comfortably enjoy
2. Pour 2-4 cups of Epsom salt into the water as it's filling up
3. Make sure the salt has been dissolved in the water before getting into the tub
4. Turn down the lights and light a single candle (optional)
5. Add 3-5 essential oil drops, like lavender, to an infuser or right into the water to further calm your nervous system and relax (optional)
6. Close your eyes, try to meditate if you'd like, or put on some relaxing music, and soak for 15 – 30 minutes
7. Towel off and if possible, try to go right to bed without any further stimulation

Once you've tried this method, I think you'll be hooked… It's one of the most relaxing spa-like experiences you can do right at home and it costs less than $1 a bath. I can't recommend it enough, even if it's just once a week!

REBOUNDING

Sticking with the theme of moving the lymphatic system, I want to introduce you to something you may have enjoyed as a child, but have long forgotten about.

Do you remember jumping up and down on a trampoline? Do you remember how fun it was to become weightless for a second mid-air before landing back down on the soft mat only to be propelled back upwards again on every jump?

Well, that same backyard playground device is now being touted for its health benefits. Only now it's being called a "rebounder." I produced a podcast on the "33 Reasons to Use a Rebounder," which detailed the many health benefits attributed to using a trampoline, which includes improved cardiovascular function, pulmonary function, blood pressure, blood sugar, weight loss, detoxification, skin improvement, and mood.

Basically, it's a scientifically proven exercise to enhance circulation and detoxification while having a lot of fun!

The nice thing is that companies have manufactured smaller 3' rebounders for home use that can be tucked away as needed. And, most brands include a bar to hold onto in case you're not sure about your balance in the beginning.

On the resource page for this book, I will link up a video to demonstrate how to use a rebounder, where to purchase one, and how often to use it.

STEAM

At the clinics in India and Sri Lanka, patients would always be brought to a steam bed or hut after their Pancha Karma massage was complete.

The patient's entire body would be exposed to steam heat, with the exception of their head. These steam devices allowed for a massive amount of perspiration within just minutes. This practice is called Swedana in Ayurvedic Medicine.

The reason you'd want to sweat after your massage is because during a massage, you've already stimulated the lymphatic fluid and began to mobilize toxins. This is the perfect time to help them safely make their way right out of the body by sweating them out. This is one of the amazing functions of your body. It knows how to cleanse and detox itself as long as it's given the proper channels and support.

Plus, too few people really break a sweat anymore. Most people don't exercise and we no longer do manual labor. This means the odds of you naturally detoxing through your sweat is severely limited. This can then lead to a further build-up of toxins in your blood and cells.

So, if you can't be out in the sun sweating during the day, I highly recommend finding another way to do so at least a few times per week. There are a few different steam and sauna options, which I will explain in a moment. Some can be done right at home, and others may be found locally at most wellness centers.

HOW TO STEAM

You probably don't need to much of an explanation on how to sweat, so I'm going to keep this simple and provide a few ways to enhance your treatment.

1. Keep the humidity at 100% to maintain moist air (steam only)
2. The temperature can be set as low as you'd like, but most steam rooms range between 70-90 Celsius and 150-200 degrees Fahrenheit (I recommend the lower end of the heat range)
3. Start at a lower temperature around 110-120F if you've never done a steam before
4. Wear just a small towel or nothing at all to allow your skin to fully breathe
5. Start with just 5-10 minutes maximum
6. Exit the steam room if you feel light-headed, dizzy, too hot, or for any other issue

(Note: Because most public steam rooms do not filter their water, poisoness chlorine gas is expelled into the air you're breathing. Therefore, I cannot recommend steam rooms that enclose your whole body unless the water has gone through a reverse osmosis filter to remove the contaminants that you'll breathing as a gas vapor.)

DETOX & BEYOND

The other benefits to steam beyond detoxification are a potential lowering of blood pressure, expectorant of mucus from your chest or sinuses, and a decrease in certain types of pain (see the sauna section next for additional details).

Sun bathing and steam sessions have been used for over 6,000 years and have remained a staple in natural healing because they work. I highly recommend choosing some modality that causes you to perspire at least a few times per week. The benefits are cumulative and your body will thank you.

SAUNA

The benefits of using a sauna are comparable to a steam room, with a few exceptions and added benefits.

A sauna, unlike the moist air of a steam, is dry heat. This is preferred by many people who like the less damp environment. The most notable differences I see in my practice is that anyone with an upper respiratory issue enjoys the expectorant effects of the steam and those with arthritis or joint pain seem to prefer the dry, desert-like, heat of the sauna.

But, as I stated, both treatments will allow you to sweat and expel toxins through your skin. Plus, there are some new and exciting studies being done with heat and its potential for improving longevity.

One of the reasons for this is because heat acts as a hermetic response that can reduce damage to the proteins in your body, as well as boosting antioxidant capacity. This allows for better recovery and tissue repair.

Saunas can also greatly reduce tension on the body and calm the nervous system. This makes it a perfect synergist to your workouts. If you're able to take a 10-20 minute dry sauna after a resistance workout, you may just find yourself recuperating much faster between workouts.

The only downside to a sauna is that it's impractical to have one at home unless you have the space for it. They also cost considerably more than an at-home steam unit because they're usually made from various types of wood and beautifully crafted.

However, I was able to find a few portable units that can fold away when not in use. The at-home option I like is by Therasage and mimics the Ayurvedic "sweat boxes" I used overseas. There are actually many options for these personal units and they can range from $300 up to over $1,000 depending on the material and technology used. I will list my top picks on the resource page.

Completing a sauna session is just like that of using a steam except there is much lower humidity. The temperature and protocol remain the same. Like with all high heat environments you may just need to work your way up in time from a few minutes during your first session to 10-20+ minutes as your body gets acclimated to the heat.[11]

THE FORGOTTEN HISTORY OF SAUNA

Before I describe the differences in using the proven effectiveness of an infrared sauna on detoxification, I wanted to share with you a history of how saunas have been used throughout the ages. A lot of times we believe we invented these new protocols, but really we're just rediscovering and improving upon them with the latest scientific advances.

Stone Age. It is believed that the first saunas were holes dug into the earth. Heated rocks were placed in the holes, then water was poured over them. Animal skins were used to cover the holes and retain the steam and humidity.

5000 - 3000 B.C. Finland: saunas were used for bathing, for childbirth, as places where a person could refresh and rejuvenate their spirits, clear their minds, and some ceremonies. Introduction of the sauna to Finland itself occurs by people who migrated from an area northwest of present day Tibet.

2000 B.C. Mayans used sweat houses for therapy and ritual.

1700 B.C. Crete: Numerous saunas appear along the Mediterranean and the world's first bathtub appears in the palace of King Minos.

1000 B.C. China: *Palm healing* is introduced as a type of healing in which one person lays their palm(s) in a healing act onto the sick person. Palms naturally radiate infrared rays.

1000 B.C. Native American sweat lodges were created as holes dug in the ground covered with a cloth. They were found in North and South America and documented with the European invasion of the Western Hemisphere.

568 B.C. The ancient medical text, *the Ayurveda*, written in Sanskrit, prescribes the sweat bath as a health measure.

500 B.C. The Greek physician, Parmenides, states that if only he had the means to create fever, he could cure all illness.

450 B.C. The historian, Herodutus, records that the Greeks have been using steam for some time to induce sweating as a form of bathing and to help maintain health.

600 – 900 A.D. Tibet: The first recorded wooden saunas were used.

1237 Batu-Khan, grandson of Genghis Khan, witnesses Russians in the winter jumping out of wooden huts, red and hot, into cold water. His aides explain to him that the secret of Russian strength is in this "exercise."

1496 German painter, Albrecht Durer, produces the illustration "The Women's Bath." It shows a scene of women in a traditional sauna washing themselves.

1567 Mexico: A history text describes Indians taking sauna baths in temescallis—low buildings large enough to fit 10 at a time.

1638 America: The Finnish-style sauna is in use in North America, brought here by the Finns. Native saunas have already long been in use by the Inuit and Native American Indian groups.

1893. USA: Dr. Kellogg introduces his electric light bath (using light bulbs as the heat source) at the 1893 World's Fair in Chicago. The heat from the light bulbs radiates much of their energy in the *far infrared range*.

1890s. Austria: Dr. Winternz brings Kellogg's invention to Europe, where he manufactures and sells 1000 infrared units, including to royalty and athletic clubs.

1920's Germany: Whole body infrared therapy comes into use by physicians in an independently developed form.

1959 NASA uses saunas to study the effects of re-entry heat on the human body.

1965 Japan: Dr. Tadashi Ishikowa, a member of the Research and Development Department of Fuji Medical, receives a patent on the zirconia ceramic infrared heater.

1965 – 1979 Japan: Medical practitioners in Japan use infrared thermal systems for healing.

1979 Japan: Infrared heaters are released for public use.

1981 – today. USA: Infrared technology becomes further refined and is sold in the United States. Refinements include modularity, new heater materials, non-toxic adhesives, large size selection, and price reduction.

1980's – Today Germany: Klinik St. Georg creates a successful cancer treatment protocol that includes hyperthermia (infrared) treatment.

Today, there is one sauna for every two to three Finns and sauna design is a revered art in Finland (and all around the world).[12]

So, as you can see, saunas have been used throughout time and we've come a long way from digging holes in the ground to now using advanced heat therapies to improve overall health and the aging process.

INFRARED SAUNA TECHNOLOGY

One of these specific advanced therapies is called, infrared (IFR) technology. Simply put, this technology mimics the rays of the sun and naturally heats the body from the inside out. This is different than regular Finnish saunas like the ones described previously.

Finnish saunas heat the ambient air around you, but not your core temperature directly. Neither one is necessarily better than the other, but the infrared benefits cannot be ascertained without this specific technology in the units.

There are also different wave lengths that allow for the infrared waves to penetrate your body at varying depths. Many people choose far infrared for detoxification, mid wave lengths for pain relief in the joints and tissues, and then near infrared for subcutaneous weight loss. However, you will get all these benefits regardless of the range you specify – they may be just more pronounced with certain settings.

Keep in mind that an infrared sauna is about 40º Fahrenheit cooler than a regular dry sauna. The reason for this is that a typical infrared sauna should last 25-minutes or more in order to get the full benefits. Therefore, the lower heat (120-150ºF) allows you to stay in longer.

IFR BENEFITS

The goal of an infrared sauna session is not necessarily to sweat profusely. Sweating may take a little longer than in a regular sauna, but the real benefit comes from allowing the infrared invisible wave technology to penetrate about 3-5mm below your skin and begin to create an increase in core temperature.

This is similar to a fever where the body can kill viruses, bacteria, and other harmful microbes. Plus, infrared saunas began to become more popular when studies showed it is possible to detoxify heavy metals like mercury from your body when using regular infrared sauna treatments.[13]

One of the most popular ways to use an infrared sauna is directly after a workout or massage. This is what I refer to as a modern-day Pancha Karma treatment. First, you get your lymphatic system mobilizing toxins by exercising or getting a massage and then the infrared sauna allows you to safely push them out through your skin.

Infrared saunas now also come with built into light therapy (chronotherapy), relaxing music, and even vibrational calming technology on the higher-end units. The directions for using an infrared sauna is pretty much the same as a steam or regular dry sauna, but with just a few exceptions:

HOW TO USE AN INFRARED SAUNA

1. Ideally, get a massage or do the "3-minute self-massage" first
2. Heat the sauna to 120-150º Fahrenheit
3. Turn on infrared panels or technology
4. Sit in sauna for 25-50 minutes
5. Safely get out of sauna sooner if you feel any adverse effects
6. Make sure you shower after an infrared sauna, or at least towel off completely to remove any heavy metals or toxins that may be on your skin after having been detoxed

Infrared saunas are steadily growing in popularity and if you're lucky you may find a wellness center in your local area that has one. Try it out for a series of 3-5 sessions within a week or two to get the most benefit. If you like it, and you think you may use it more often, it may be a worthwhile investment in your health.

To find my updated recommendations go to: StephenCabral.com/rbe

DENTAL AMALGAMS

I feel like I would be doing you a disservice if I didn't include a small excerpt on the health issues that can come from improper dental care.

So often, I find that many doctors do not even look in a patient's mouth to assess their oral health. One of the reasons why this is a must is to look for any potential causes of their symptoms. As I sated earlier in the book, inflammation or infections in your mouth can actually lead to a shortened lifespan and other health issues.

My highest recommendation is to seek out a holistic or biological dentist that specializes in and is certified in mercury amalgam removal and holistic dentistry. It typically does not cost any more money out pocket, but you'll get far more benefit from their knowledge and experience in natural oral health.

ORAL HEALTH ISSUES TO LOOK FOR:

- Inflammation (redness and puffiness) of the gums
- Discoloration of gums, teeth, or lips
- Gingivitis
- Plaque or tartar build up
- Bacterial infections (pus)
- Heavy metal implants
- Mercury/silver amalgams
- Multiple metals in your mouth ("silver," gold, etc.)
- Old root canals (they may have hidden infections under them)

Please also keep in mind that if your mercury amalgams need to be removed, I recommend that your body is healthy and strong enough to do so before planning this removal.

You will also need to be doing a 1-3 week pre-removal detox protocol, as well as another 3 weeks post-removal. Using an infrared sauna the day and weeks following your mercury amalgam removal is recommended. I will enclose my 3-week protocol for anyone looking to detox their body for all health reasons in the last part to this book.

Here is a website to find a holistic dentist in your area:

https://iabdm.org/location/

COFFEE ENEMAS

Coffee and enemas aren't usually two words that are used together…

And although most people aren't familiar with this type of detoxification protocol, they've actually been used for quite some time. Believe it or not, they were in the Merck medical handbook up until the 1970's and used throughout World War II for pain management.[14]

Today, coffee enemas are used in natural cancer treatment centers all across the world for their renowned ability to boost your body's most powerful cancer fighting antioxidant called glutathione (s-transferase). Glutathione is often referred to as the "mother of all antioxidants" and is naturally produced by your liver to help keep you healthy.[15]

By doing a coffee enema, you are dramatically enhancing your liver's own natural detoxification ability. Again, this is why natural cancer treatment and other holistic wellness centers use coffee enemas so frequently. Coffee enemas also help to decrease your chances of feeling any Herxheimer reactions ("die-off") if you're detoxing from a major health issue. This treatment allows your liver to dump toxins straight into your intestines and expel them right out of your body when you have a bowel movement following the enema.

This whole process takes places by simply giving yourself an emema using an organic caffeinated coffee. When the coffee enters your rectum, it moves up your colon and through the hepatic portal duct to your liver. Your liver then dilates the thousands of bile ducts contained within it and stimulates the detoxification process.

After just a few minutes of circulating the coffee through your colon and liver, the body already begins to detox. It's amazing how such a simple process using an all-natural food based product can help improve your health so much. Enemas have also been used as far back as 6,000 years ago in Ayurvedic medicine (called "Basti") and they're even talked about in the Bible.

Now before you begin to think you couldn't possibly give yourself a coffee enema, I want to share with you how painless and easy a process it really is.

COFFEE ENEMAS MADE SIMPLE

1. Brew 3 TBSP of organic caffeinated coffee with 1000ml of distilled or filtered water in a French press coffee maker (or boiling water in a pot)
2. Allow the coffee to brew for 10 minutes
3. Press down the French Press and then let the coffee cool to room temperature
4. Pour the 1000ml of coffee into the stainless-steel enema bucket (ensure the sterile tubes are already attached and clamped closed)
5. Place the bucket on a table approximately 3' above the ground
6. Place a towel down and lie on your back.
7. Insert the small thin part of the tub about 3-6" into your rectum. (Use an oil or gel to lubricate the tube)

8. Unlock the clamp and allow the coffee to begin to slowly flow into your body.
9. After all the coffee has been emptied from the bucket, turn over onto your right side (do not remove the tube, since it can cause a release of the liquid back out of your body).
10. Try to hold the coffee in for 12-15 minutes by breathing and relaxing your body. Read a book or listen to music to distract yourself if needed.
11. When you need to release the coffee enema from your body simply sit on the toilet and allow all of the liquid to be expelled.

The amazing science behind coffee enemas is that the speed of blood flow through the liver is enhanced, which allows you to clean all the blood in your body every 3-6 minutes. With boosted antioxidant capacity this creates a supercharge for your liver to take its natural ability to the next level.

If you're currently dealing with a major health issue, where more intense detoxification protocols are warranted, I highly recommend looking more into the benefits of coffee enemas. The Gerson Institute has quite a bit of information on them. And, if you're already feeling pretty good an occasional coffee enema can help you maintain your clean and happy body.

THE DR. CABRAL DETOX HOUR

By now, I'm sure you're starting to see how beneficial some of these detox treatments can be, but often the question then comes up as to how to put it all together…

To make it easy, I've created a straight-forward protocol for you to follow. This simple, but powerful home detox treatment can be completed in just 60-minutes. It includes one lymphatic treatment, a steam or sauna session, and then a coffee enema. This is literally a modern-day Pancha Karma treatment you can do right at home to get well, drop the weight, and live longer!

HERE HOW TO COMPLETE IT:

First, choose from the dry brushing, self-massage, or rebounding options above. Any of these 3 will begin to get your lymphatic fluid moving and prepare you to push those toxins safely out of the body.
(5-10 minutes)

Second, choose from a steam, sauna, or infrared sauna. This will enable you to easily sweat out those mobilized toxins from your body.
(20-40 minutes)

Finally, after you towel off from your sauna, you can begin your coffee enema that should have already cooled down to room temperature if you brewed it before you started this modern-day detox protocol.
(15-20 minutes)

You can complete this healing "Dr. Cabral Detox Hour" once a week or even just once a month to enjoy the hundreds of benefits associated with enhanced wellness and a dramatic emptying of your rain barrel!

ADDITIONAL TOXIC REMOVAL BENEFITS

Although I mainly spoke about the powerful detoxifying benefits of the treatments above, they are highly beneficial in dozens of other areas.

Some of those areas include:

- Improved blood pressure
- Increased arterial function of the heart
- Cellulite reduction
- Skin rejuvenation
- Decreased digestive stress
- Enhanced energy
- Pain reduction

I hope this chapter opened and expanded your mind to additional possibilities that you may not be including in your life right now, but can now use to improve your overall well-being and vitality!

And as I stated before, instead of having this be a 700-page book, I've included the additional details, recommendations, up to date product links, etc. on the resource page at: StephenCabral.com/rbe

In the next chapter, I can't wait to compliment all these healing detox treatments we just reviewed with the new science of upgraded rest and relaxation!

HOW TO EMPTY YOUR RAIN BARREL™ BY MANUALLY REMOVING TOXINS

At the end of each chapter, I try to include one action plan item to implement that I believe will give you the most "bang for your buck." As a big believer in the 80/20 rule, I know that a few small changes can make a big difference in your life.

Because of that, I am recommending you choose dry brushing over the other treatments to start. If you can do them all or more than one, then that's great… However, in my practice the one that most people seem to be able to stick with on a near daily basis is dry brushing.

Dry brushing takes all of 3-minutes every morning or before you get in the shower, and it's so simple to do. It's also easy to travel with, and you can feel the benefits immediately. It's my top pick for draining and moving the lymphatic system.

Simply follow the steps I've outlined on the previous pages for how to dry brush your body for maximum effectiveness – But remember, as long as you're gently stroking with the brush towards your heart you really can't go wrong!

Rest

I have a confession to make.

In my ideal world, I would never sleep. Yes, you heard that right…

I'd much prefer to split my daytime hours helping people in my practice and enjoying time with my family. At night, when everyone else sleeps, I'd like to catch up on more reading, watching movies, doing research, and writing my next book.

I've had to fight this yearning for more "life" my whole life. And the issue was that even when I felt healthy in late 20s, I was still missing one crucial item if I hoped to ever maintain that state: sleep.

So, starting at 27 years old, I made sleep, rest, and shutting down my body for a period of time a priority.

For me, this meant creating a sleep schedule, getting rid of my insomnia, and finding time to "do nothing" (more on this *nothingness* later). Back then, it was easier said than done, but I had a big "why," and that was to never live another day as that sick kid that missed out on a lot of years of his life.

The truth is that rest and sleep are so much more important than we give them credit for. The reason for this is that until you calm your body down and switch into the parasympathetic (rest and repair) side of your nervous system, you're most likely stuck in fight or flight mode.[1]

Although the sympathetic nervous system (the fight or flight side) can make you feel energized and productive, it can burn you out. In this chapter, I'm going to show you how to balance both sides of your nervous system so that you can naturally increase your energy levels, alertness, concentration, and clarity of thinking, while simultaneously improving your digestion, hormones, inflammation, and waist line...

Let's first start with your energy levels.

BROKEN RHYTHMS

Much of the world right now pays very little attention to the natural rhythms of the world around them, and therefore, they pay little attention to their own built in alarm clock.

What I mean by this is that every human works on what's called a circadian diurnal rhythm, which in a perfect state allows you to wake up (without an alarm clock) as the sun rises and start to get tired as the sun sets. That is exactly how human biology is supposed to work.

As the sun rises, our cortisol levels begin to rise along with it, and then as the day progresses our cortisol levels gradually decline. Ultimately, our cortisol levels should be almost zero around 10:00pm. This is crucial for helping us to begin the repair process inside our body. The setting sun also triggers melatonin to be produced, which helps us get into a deep sleep.[2]

NORMAL CORTISOL CURVE

Keep in mind, the graph above depicts an *ideal* cortisol rhythm and oftentimes what I see in my practice is dysfunctional diurnal rhythms leading to the big 3 energy health issues. Below, I review those 3 energy and nervous system dysfunctions and why they need to be corrected for both body and mind well-being.

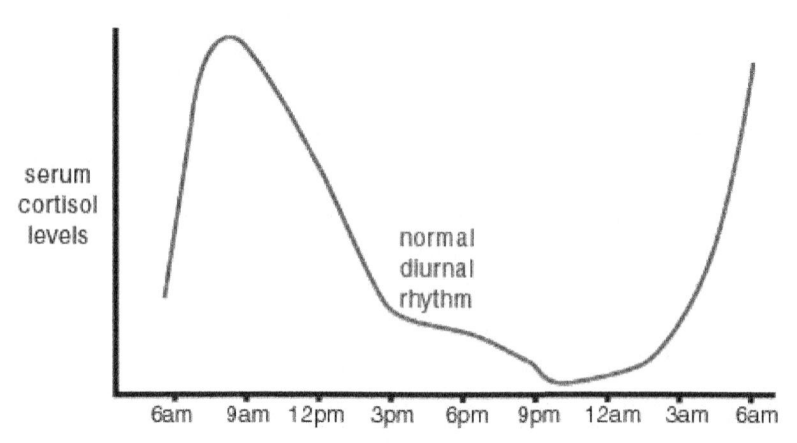

(The graph above depicts energy (cortisol) levels peaking shortly after waking and slowly lowering throughout the day. By 10:00pm cortisol levels are at their lowest and this is why going to bed by 9-10pm is essential for long-term health)

WIRED (HIGH CORTISOL)

Although I see someone new each week suffering from adrenal fatigue or energy issues, I very rarely see someone in the "wired" state.

The wired state is when you literally feel like you can go-go-go all day, take on dozens of different projects, and need very little sleep to get by. You may actually not even be really sleeping at all, since you can't turn off your racing mind . . .

As I said, very few people come to me in this state, since they actually believe they have plenty of energy and they are doing great. Plus, they've already overbooked themselves and are too busy juggling school, work, or family to make anytime to slow down!

These "wired puppies" are working off pure adrenaline and cortisol. The way you can always tell the difference between natural energy and wired energy is that someone with natural energy isn't anxious and can actually sit down and do nothing. Wired puppies can't slow down, sit down, and be happy without moving.

Here's what their adrenal cortisol rhythm looks like (Cushing's disease is the extreme of an exaggerated high cortisol output):

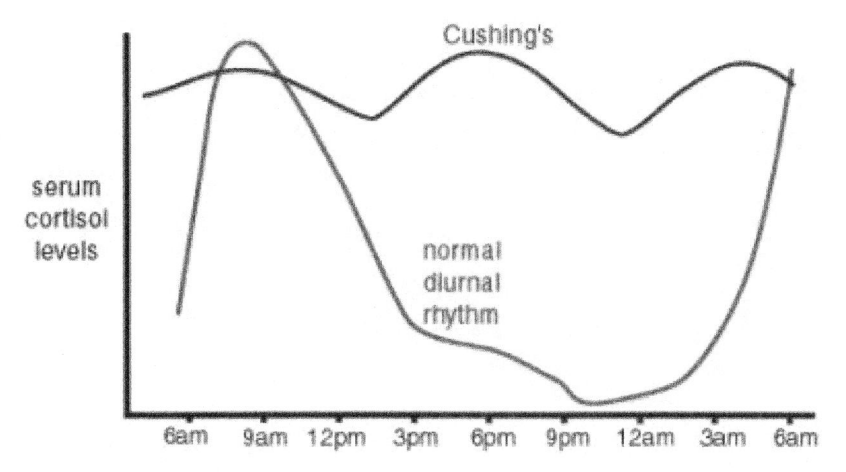

(The top line in the graph above is depicting someone with extreme cortisol output, referred to as Cushing's disease. People suffering from Cushing's or even just high cortisol output often have terrible insomnia, anxiety, and other disorders stemming from this "wired" state induced by high cortisol secretion from the adrenal glands.)

Now, I know many with burn out and/or adrenal fatigue (CFS) would love to have that much cortisol streaming through their veins, but I can assure you it's not a good thing and it does eventually lead to burn out, as well as a host of other possible health issues such as Alzheimer's, dementia, heart disease, high blood pressure, digestive issues, estrogen dominant symptoms, autoimmune dis-eases, and much more…

So, if you or anyone you know is stuck in this "wired" state, please seek help before you end up in our next stage called "Tired & Wired."

TIRED & WIRED UPSIDE DOWN CORTISOL CURVE

Feeling "tired and wired" is a classic case of adrenal resistance. This means your HPA axis is getting burnt out and your hypothalamus, pituitary gland and adrenals (HPA) are not able to keep up with the stress demands you are placing on them. As a result, you produce less cortisol from the adrenal glands when you wake up.

And since cortisol is one of your natural get-up-and-go energy sources, you wake up feeling a little groggy, and slow to get moving – Which is why you may reach for coffee or caffeine to artificially spike your tired adrenals to "squeeze out" more cortisol.

But, the biggest problem of all with the tired and wired adrenal dysfunction state is that although you feel tired during the day, you may actually get an energy spike at night when it's time to wind down for bed!

Basically, you feel like you could sleep all day and stay up all night. This is, of course, a recipe for burn out. Here's what it looks like on a graph:

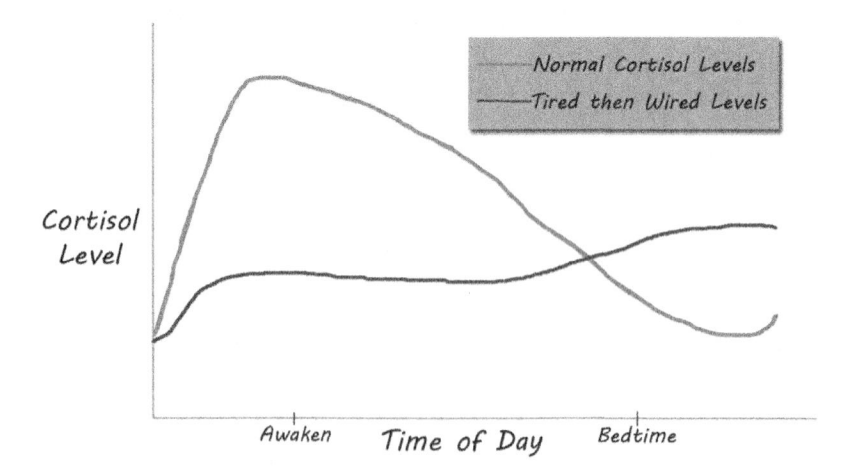

(The image above of the bottom line shows a low morning cortisol rise and a higher evening time energy spike making getting up difficult and falling or staying asleep challenging. Image source: tetonsage.com)

The tired and wired stage is oftentimes where I see people come into my practice with their first complaints of fatigue, poor sleep patterns, aches, pains, brain fog, memory loss, hormone imbalances, blood sugar dysregulation, and lowered metabolism.

If you don't take care of your adrenal and HPA Axis health at this point you may just end up in our last stage.

TIRED ALL THE TIME (LOW CORTISOL)

The last stage of adrenal fatigue is true burn out, but from a much deeper level. When you hit this rock bottom state, not even a good nap, a week of great sleeping, or a month's vacation is enough to bring your energy levels back.

You have all-day brain fog, your joints or muscles most likely hurt, you have no energy, and your immune system is now faltering…

It's at this stage, where you know that something is wrong. Exercise, eating, and even going out to dinner seem like big tasks. You feel anxious, overwhelmed, irritable, and you just want to spend time alone resting. It's not a great way to live.

MY STRUGGLE WITH ADRENAL FATIGUE

Unfortunately, I ended up here at 17 years old. I was at the opposite end of Cushing's Disease. I was actually diagnosed Addison's Disease after completing an ACTH simulation test that showed I was no longer producing adequate levels of cortisol.

I wasn't happy to get this diagnosis, but at least I now knew why even slight exertion sent me into a month-long ear/nose/throat sickness and swollen glands. Many people don't realize this, but you need norepinephrine and cortisol to regulate inflammation, other hormones, and your immune system. I lacked that lever, and it made life very unpleasant.

Although most people will never get to this point, having lowered levels of cortisol literally makes you feel like you have less "life" in you. It's a terrible feeling to be so tired that you don't even want to speak, go out with friends, or even think about planning a vacation.

All you want to do is hide-away and be by yourself and do nothing. I believe this state is *not* indicative of a mental disorder, but rather a protective biological function of your body wanting you to stay clear of any stress that could wipe it out further. However, the cold conventional medicine perspective initially labeled me as depressed and that my complaints were "all in my head."

Here's what the tired all the time cortisol rhythm looks like:

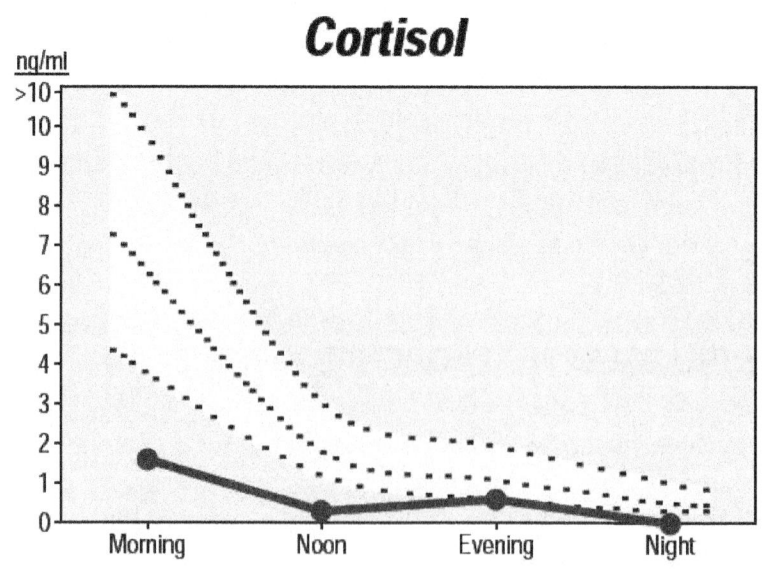

Cortisol

(The image above of the bottom bolded line shows low cortisol output all day long versus the normal variants or the dotted-line cortisol range.)

The good news is this:

No matter what stage you're at, any level of fatigue can be overcome. You can get your energy, stamina, libido, drive, ambition, and mental clarity back.

It all starts with Emptying Your Rain Barrel™ through this DESTRESS Protocol™. In this particular instance, you absolutely must take back your sleep and rest time.

To this day, I can tell you that the most important thing I did to repair my HPA Axis and chronic fatigue immune dysfunction syndrome (CFIDS) was to create a sleep schedule.

I know that seems obvious after what you just read, but to be honest, the information I just shared with you isn't taught in this way to medical and health professionals. That's why it's so hard to be diagnosed in the first place.

(Side Note: You can run this same at-home adrenal saliva test if you'd like to test your own cortisol and hormone levels to see what stage of adrenal output you're at. Go to StephenCabral.com/rbe for details.)

We all want more energy in the morning and we want to be able to fall asleep at night (and stay asleep). To do this we must first take back control of our sleeping patterns.

Once you get your sleep pattern in order, you will have taken the first step to allowing your body to naturally produce the energy hormones and neurotransmitters you need during the first part of the day, and the calming sleep hormones, etc. you need at night to fall into a deep restorative sleep.

Hopefully, you now understand the vital importance of regulating your body's rhythm to match your natural cortisol and melatonin production, so let's get right into how you can maximize your rest and sleep cycles.

MY TOP 3 WAYS TO RESET YOUR SLEEP
30-MINUTE RULE

In order to get your body to naturally produce the chemicals it needs to wake up and fall asleep without assistance, you need to push it back into a rhythm. The best way to do this is to go to bed within 30-minutes of the same time each day – 7 days a week.

Literally, one of the major reasons why I'm now able to wake up with boundless energy (without caffeine) is because I made myself start waking up at 6:00am every day. Some days, it's 5:30am, and on the weekends, it's never later than 6:30am. Believe it or not, waking up at this time everyday gives me more energy – not less!

The reason for this is that, I'm now tired by 9:00pm and want to go to bed around 9:30-10:00pm nightly. So, by getting into bed no later than 10:00pm each night, I can fall right to sleep and wake up 7.5-8 hours later naturally without an alarm clock.

Eventually, your body will be locked into such a perfect sleep rhythm that you'll be able to have a late night or early morning without any side effects. I just recommend giving yourself at least 21 days to initially get into a sleep cycle.

10-6

No human is a night owl.

But, this is no longer a common-sense statement, and I debate this all the time with well-intentioned health practitioners who believe that some people "naturally" do produce more cortisol and energy at night.

Unfortunately, those health practitioners do not understand the innate circadian rhythms that all humans are born with as demonstrated in the graphs above. (The one exception to this rule are people whom are sight-impaired that are not always able to create a typical diurnal rhythm due to the inability to see all of the sun's spectrum of light rays.)

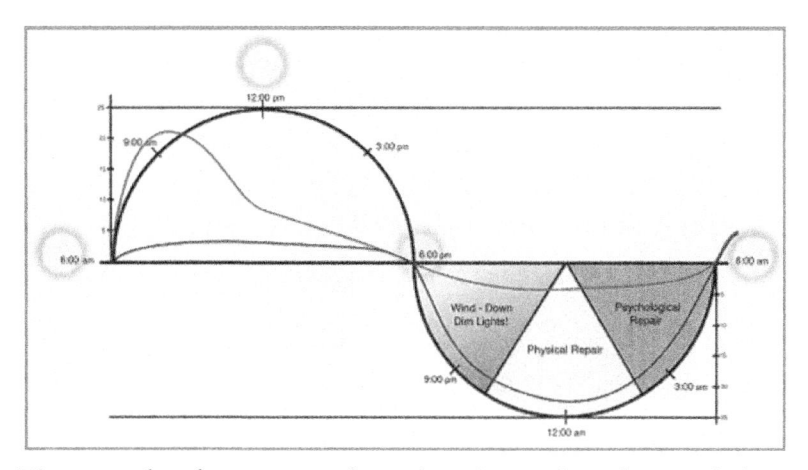

(This is one of my favorite images for teaching the true diurnal energy rhythm we are looking to create within the body. From 6:00am - 6:00pm we are meant to experience ups and downs in stress and energy output, and then from 6:00pm - 6:00am we should be winding down, limiting our exposure to light, and sleeping for about 8 hours to allow for repair, detoxification, and rejuvenation to happen.)

As you can see from the image above, melatonin (your sleep hormone) is in direct opposition to cortisol. If you're stressed, exposed to bright light, or working late, you lose the cancer-fighting and sleep inducing benefits of this powerful hormone, melatonin.

Night owls believe they do their best work at night. This is a "wired" or "tired & wired" dysfunction and one that can be corrected within 1-2 weeks by removing all electronics, lights, and creating a natural sleep environment.

I know this seems funny to say, but I if you were to go live in the woods for 3 weeks you'd automatically reset your wake/sleep cycle. Without blinds on your windows or electricity to keep lights on at night you wouldn't be able to create the artificial environment that allows you to be a night owl. Within weeks of waking up to the sunlight around 6:00am, you'd be so tired at night, you'd begin to go to bed earlier naturally as the sun sets.

This brings me to my next point. The closer you go to bed when it gets dark out and closer you wake up to when the sun rises the more natural energy you will have. You will now be working with your own innate rhythms, which are eternally connected with nature. For most people in my practice, the best compromise we can get to is going to bed between 9:30-10:30pm and then waking up 8 hours later – about 5:30-6:30am.

In the long run, the more hours you're in bed asleep before midnight, the better, since you'll be taking advantage of your built-in circadian rhythm of breaking down your body during the day (catabolism) and repairing it at night (anabolism).

(Note: I do understand that some people have to work the overnight shift, or may not be able to go to bed by 10:00pm and wake up at 6:00am.)

Although working the night shift has been proven to be less healthy due to a lack of melatonin production, etc.,[3] you still can be healthy if you create some type of daily rhythm where you're going to bed at the same time and waking up 8 hours later each day.)

THE 15-MINUTE METHOD

Now that you know, sleeping from approximately 10:00pm – 6:00am is the most natural rhythm for your body to get into, the next question usually is, "how can I get to bed that early?!"

Many people come to me, with a bedtime of somewhere around 12:00am/midnight. I let them know that eventually that really should be worked backwards. It truly is that important if you want to Empty Your Rain Barrel™ of stress, fat accumulation, and toxins, as well as boost beneficial hormone production. Luckily, the remedy to the late to bed, late to rise problem is quite simple…

The easiest way to reset your sleep schedule is to simply move your current bed-time back by 15-minutes each week.

By using this strategy, your brain and body won't fight or even notice the subtle changes taking place. It's the same type of methodology I use for weaning people of high-doses of caffeine. By getting into bed 15-minutes earlier every night, this will also allow you to wake up 15-minutes earlier.

Some people decide to just change their sleep cycle all at once and deal with a few tired days while resetting, but the "15-Minute Method" is a gentler approach that works well – and it allows you to find what time is the most realistic for you to get to bed and wake up.

Perhaps you'll never be the 9:30/10:00pm bed time person, but even going to bed an hour earlier will dramatically improve your melatonin and cortisol rhythms, which will then benefit your health, waist line, and longevity.

10 TIPS FOR SOUNDER SLEEP

The 3 tips above will help you improve your overall sleep cycle, but now I'd also like to help you actually get to sleep faster and stay asleep longer, so here are my favorite tips I've successfully used myself and with thousands of others:

1. STOP EATING 2-3 HOURS BEFORE BED

Eating right before bed can actually make it harder to fall sleep since you'll be producing more energy for digestion. Plus, when you go to bed, you want your body to focus on rejuvenation, repair, and detoxification – not on digesting the last meal in your stomach. Remember, it's difficult for autophagy (detox and cancer fighting) to take place if there is no down-time where no new toxins are coming in.

2. MAKE YOUR ROOM PITCH BLACK

If you live in the city, like I do, the city lights make it difficult to produce enough melanopsin, which then creates melatonin since it's triggered by the sun setting and the invisible blue light seen by your retinas at that time.[4]

That's why black out shades and blinds make such a *huge* difference. An ideal bedroom for sleep is so dark you can't see your hand 3-feet in front of you. This ensures you will be setting yourself up for adequate sleep hormones to be produced.

Blue-blocking sunglass companies also make glasses to use at night if you must continue to use your phone or computer within an hour or two of bed. These glasses help to block the light rays that decrease melatonin and increase cortisol.

3. WAKE UP TO LIGHT

You may have already guessed this as the next step, but if darkness helps produce more melatonin, then light forces it to decrease. This is exactly what you want in order to wake up naturally without the grogginess.

The problem is that if you're using black-out shades and blinds to block light from coming in, you're also going to inhibit the morning sun rise light from touching your eyelids and skin.

This is what used to happen to me and although I'd fall asleep fine, I'd wake up groggy due to a lack of light from the sun to wake me up naturally. I was rescued from this dilemma completely when I discovered the "wake-light."

This remarkable feat of technology actually allows you to set an alarm clock to your desired wake time, and then about 30-minutes before that desired wake time the wake-light begins to get brighter each minute for 30-minutes until you wake up naturally. And if for some reason you don't wake up peacefully by just the light alone, the alarm clock begins to gradually play the sounds of birds chirping…

This wake-light alarm clock really is as great as it sounds and it doubles as a fantastic way to fight Seasonal Affective Disorder (SAD), or low mood during the darker months of the year.

(Note: Light Box Therapy can also be tremendous for SAD and only needs to be done for about 30-minutes upon waking.)

4. COOL DOWN

The ideal temperature in a room for the best sleeping conditions is 67-69 degrees (Fahrenheit). Cooler is okay, but warmer is not recommended. Your body temperature should naturally decrease as you go to sleep, and lying in a hot room can disrupt sleep.

A few hours before bed, try to turn down the thermostat in your bedroom and just add another blanket to the foot of the bed if you end up needing it during the night.

Although I do not like a lot of electronic or plug-in devices near you while sleeping, some people do like various "chili pads" that actually cool the bed while you sleep. These are excellent for couples that prefer different temperatures in bed. I recommend looking for a non-electronic or low/no-EMF version of these cooling pads.

5. BREATHABLE SHEETS & COVERS

Too many people (including babies) are sleeping on toxic sheets that have been dyed with chemicals and sprayed with flame retardants. These toxins can seep right into our bloodstream through contact with the skin.

Look for natural fabrics like organic cotton, bamboo, or wool. These fabrics will also allow your skin to breathe at night, which is essential for proper detoxification through your skin.

For those with allergies, purchasing dust covers for your pillows and mattress can be life-changing. These dust covers prevent dust mites from coming out from inside your mattress or pillows and onto your skin causing allergic reactions. I also recommend washing your sheets at least once per week in hot water to remove additional environmental toxins and allergens you bring in on your hair and skin from the outside.

My favorite sheets right now are made from bamboo, which is environmentally sustainable and eco-friendly. They're also naturally non-toxic, and feel 3 degrees cooler than cotton variations. To date, I've never slept on anything more soft and comfortable than these sheets!

6. WHITE NOISE

Sometimes city noise or even just complete quiet can keep you awake or lying there restless at night. To balance this white noise machines can drown out ambient sounds and help you doze off faster.

Smartphone apps and other devices typically include nature sounds like rain falling, or a running stream. Experiment with a few white noise sounds until you find one that just serves as gentle background noise that you don't even notice when it's time to sleep. If you're using your phone, just remember to set it to "airplane" mode to cut down on EMFs and WI-FI signals.

7. ELECTRONIC-FREE ZONE

One of the issues we've run into in our modern-day tech-focused culture is that we're constantly being stimulated by screens beaming light into our eyes.

Your bedroom should really be electronics-free. No TV, laptops, phone, tablets, etc. You must begin to associate your bed with sleep – not work or TV time, which will stimulate your brain wave activity. This can increase the fight/flight response and activate the HPA Axis inducing adrenaline and cortisol responses.[5]

Sleep, sex, and reading are the only activities I recommend you associate with your bed. The reason this is important is because this association will begin to create mental anchors within your brain that will trigger conditioned responses when you get into bed. It will ultimately allow you to fall asleep faster and get into a deeper, more restorative sleep.

8. WIND DOWN

About 30-minutes before bed, I recommend beginning to wind down.

This means, turn off the electronics, get yourself ready for bed, and creating your to-do list. The creation of a to-do list for tomorrow allows you to Empty Your Rain Barrel™ of all of the topics that race through your mind while lying in bed preventing you from falling into a deep relaxed state.

Simply plan-out your next day hour-by-hour and you'll begin to see how you really can take control of your life. This is an amazing tool for self-empowerment and does wonders for anxiety. There's also now no need to keep these "mental notes" running through your mind after writing them down. This one action allows you to take a deep breath and realize you've got everything accounted for on your to-do list.

(Note: Topics and tips like this are covered in much more depth on my daily free podcast, The "Cabral Concept." Check out it out on iTunes or at StephenCabral.com/podcasts)

One other item I recommend is doing 5-minutes of stretching or meditation combined with relaxed belly breathing before bed.

It can be as simple as dimming the lights, sitting on the floor, closing your eyes, breathing deeply into your belly (not chest), and completing a few seated stretches for your hips and hamstrings. This will calm your brain and nervous system enabling you to shut down your "engine" and turn off your racing mind.

9. NO NAPPING

Napping can help or hurt depending on what stage of health you've found yourself in.

If you're not a great sleeper and haven't gotten into a natural 8-hour rhythm as explained above, then I can't recommend a mid-afternoon nap just yet (even for adrenal fatigue).

The reason I say this is that although you may be tired, napping can throw of your circadian rhythm and downgrade your sleep at night when it's most needed for repair.

However, if your sleep pattern has been re-established and you're resting well at night, then an after-lunch nap can help calm the sympathetic nervous system, improve digestion, and rejuvenate the body. If you do decide to nap keep it to under 40-minutes (ideally 20-30) and always before 2:00pm if your bed-time is close to 10:00pm.

So, although I don't recommend napping until you've gotten your sleep cycle under control, I do recommend an afternoon "siesta" for everyone when possible.

This is simply a period of time post-lunch to calm your nervous system, and allow for maximum nutrient absorption, while turning off the stress of the day and shifting into the parasympathetic nervous system.

10. SUPPLEMENTS

Good quality nutritional supplements can improve most aspects of your life, and sleep is no exception.

As a former medicated insomniac who relied on Ambien, Lunesta, and Benadryl on a nightly basis to fall asleep, I can assure you there is a better way. By using the tips I provided above in addition to natural sleep aids you'll be able to reset your sleep cycle – typically within 2-3 weeks.

Also, by using Functional Medicine testing you can actually see if it's a cortisol, neurotransmitter, melatonin, or other nutrient imbalance preventing you from falling or staying asleep.

If you decide not to do an at-home Functional Medicine test, I have provided the top 3 nutritional supplements to help reset your sleep cycle.

3 SUPPLEMENTS FOR SLEEP

The nutritional supplements I'm recommending help your body by rebalancing the 3 main reasons why a person can't sleep:

1. High cortisol/stress
2. Lack of melatonin production
3. Mineral deficiencies

It's amazing the dramatic turn arounds people can have when they use this *Deep Sleep Package* to help create the natural 8-hour sleep rhythm they've been working towards. Here are the 3 supplements, that I've seen have the most impact in people's lives:

MAGNESIUM CITRATE

This form of magnesium gets into the body fast. Therefore, it is ideal to take it 30-minutes before bed as a powder in warm water or as a hot tea. Since magnesium is often missing to a great degree in people's diet, this natural mineral supplement aids the body in calming the nervous system – which then allows you to unwind and relax.

HERBAL SLEEP FORMULA

In my practice, I use an herbal formula that includes scientifically proven herbs like ashwagandha, chamomile, valerian, and passionflower. These herbs (especially ashwagandha) can act as adaptogens and calm elevated levels of cortisol naturally.

MELATONIN

Many patients and doctors don't know that melatonin is largely produced in the gut as a downline product of serotonin.

This is why there's a direct connection between intestinal G.I. issues, leaky gut, depression, and poor sleep. If you're not producing adequate serotonin because of a gut dysfunction, then you won't manufacture enough melatonin. This can prevent you from achieving the level of restorative sleep you're looking for.

In the short-term there are two different forms of melatonin I may recommend. The first one is fast acting and it's a sublingual liquid (or lozenge) you place under your tongue. It works within 20-30 minutes and gets right into your blood stream to help you fall asleep faster.

The second form of melatonin is called, prolonged release melatonin. I'll sometimes use this form when someone in my practice tells me they can fall asleep fine, but can't stay asleep. The prolonged-release melatonin is made in a tablet form that allows it to be slowly released over the period of a few hours instead of right away.

Typically, I'll use this entire sleep protocol with someone for about 2-3 weeks until we've created a sufficient sleep cycle. We'll then wean off each product by cutting the dosage in half (one product at a time) and watch how the body responds.

You may find that you begin to experience poor sleep after removing just one product. At this time, your body is simply letting you know it doesn't have enough reserves, or it's not strong enough, or balanced on its own yet to do without that nutritional supplement.

You may try to wean off whatever supplement your body needs in another 3-4 weeks again when your body gets even stronger from the synergistic DESTRESS Protocols™ you've been following.

(Note: The example above is exactly how nutritional supplements were intended to be used. Some people deem them bad or good. No such attributes need to be attributed. Supplements are there to support a body that is not quite strong enough to do it on its own, or it suffers from an imbalance in some way. Once the body is re-balanced then specialty supplements, such as those for sleeping may not be necessary – your body will ultimately let you know.)

THE SLEEP TRAP

Keep in mind that no one is perfect.

It's rare that anyone gets a perfect night of sleep every week or month of the year. The goal then should not to be perfect, but rather to get as close to perfect sleep as you can. I personally work with a lot of Type A personalities (myself included) that get upset when their sleep wasn't exactly 8 hours, their "sleep tracker app" was off, or they went to bed too late.

This type of thinking will only lead to more stress and anxiety around sleep, and ultimately prevent you from relaxing – which is what you need to do in order to get the quality sleep you desire. My advice is to simply breathe, relax, and do the best you can to get to bed earlier and wake up at the same time each morning. It took me a couple of months to fully master this. In time, it just gets easier to implement all of these healthy DESTRESS Protocols™ because we enjoy the benefit of perspective and results. It is those positive results that keep us wanting more, and therefore, create self-fulfilling healthy-lifestyle actions.

I hope you enjoyed these tried and true methods for calming your body's nervous systems and allowing you to begin to heal and repair. In the next chapter, I'd like to show you how to maximize these results using an often overlooked aspect of mind-body healing…

EMPTY YOUR RAIN BARREL™ WITH ENHANCED REST

Although there are so many things you can do to calm your central nervous system to enhance the deep healing and repair process that happens while you sleep, my highest recommendation is to begin with creating a sleep cycle.

CREATE YOUR OWN SLEEP CYCLE

The easiest way to do this is to follow my tips from this chapter and begin to work your current bed-time back by 15-minutes until you're in bed by 9:00-10:00pm. Then, allow yourself to stay in bed for ideally 8-9 hours until 5:00-7:00am.

If your work schedule does not allow for this sleep schedule, do the best you can to get 8 hours of straight sleep.

To fall asleep faster, use the supplement products I recommended, as well as some light stretching, meditation, or other calming practice such as reading fiction.

Making a to-do list to plan out your next day will also calm your racing mind and allow you to turn if off without having to worry about remembering something for that next day.

Also, if you wake up groggy, I can't recommend anything more highly than using a "wake light." This will greatly improve mood and seasonal affective disorder as well as decrease morning brain fog and grogginess.

Sleep well, my friend!

For my updated product recommendations on blue-blocker sunglasses, wake-lights, light boxes, cooling pads, sleep trackers, nutritional supplements, my favorite sheets, and much more go to: StephenCabral.com/rbe

Toxic Emotions

Talking about emotions is a tricky topic.

The reason being, there is no clinical standard measure for your state of emotional balance.

Nor is there a standard test to gauge your degree of anxiety, enlightenment, depression, happiness, sadness, etc.

Even measuring biomarkers like dopamine, serotonin, and norepinephrine can have their own drawbacks, since a low level for one person may be excellent for another. This also makes a standard of care challenging.

To make matters worse, you may even be grappling with the idea of "What is real happiness?" – or wonder if anyone can possibly dictate what another's level of happiness should be at any one given time.

MIXED EMOTIONS

In our modern day version of mental health, we've been led to believe that if we are not happy 24/7, then there must be something wrong with us…

Apparently, we've forgotten that life is meant to be an ebb and flow of emotions. Some are positive and some negative. Almost none remain neutral due to our judging, survival-based cast of mind.

When you go back and study all ancient philosophies, you also see that we can't even experience bliss, joy, or happiness, without knowing despair, anger, and sadness. One does not exist without the other.

I mention this because I want you to know it's okay to have a bad day – or even a bad week. But we seem to have forgotten this. Often, I've been working with someone in my practice and they are feeling great again for some time, they'll often email me saying they had a bad day.

I'll enquire asking what about their day was so bad? And they'll typically mention they had less energy or just felt kind of down. Whenever I read these emails or hear these statements in my clinic – this is actually when I know *they're fully well again…*

CREATING A NEW NORMAL

This is usually when I just sit back and smile. I know that their body is now so healthy that they can even recognize when they have a little less energy or their mood is down. This means that their *new normal* is state of happiness, energy and vibrancy.

When I tell them this there is typically a great realization – the lightbulb goes on and they know what I mean.

They remember just a few months back when they suffered both mentally and physically from the pain of certain issues that had plagued them for years. Now that the pain had been relieved they could actually feel when they had an *off* day…

I then explain that it is perfectly normal and healthy to feel a little low at times. Maybe you've been stressed at work, you've been getting less sleep, your relationship isn't where it should be, or you're weighed down with another physical/emotional issue.

Whatever the cause, our emotions can greatly affect our physical health. And although an off day or two here or there is perfectly acceptable, when those days begin to add up and you find yourself feeling consistently down, you may have a chronic emotional problem that is the real factor impacting your physical well-being.

Often depression, anxiety, panic attacks, OCD, PTSD, and other mental imbalances hold us back from truly enjoying the life we were meant to live. So, if you suffer from more than just the occasional low mood day, I'd like to help you first recognize what may be the underlying root cause of these emotions, and then talk about how you can Empty Your Rain Barrel™ so you can be truly happy again. This will then allow you to live the life you've always wanted.

You deserve to be happy, let's show you how –

LISTEN TO YOUR EMOTIONS

I discovered these next 9 emotional triggers just a few years back and I've found identifying them incredibly helpful as a starting point – I hope you do as well.

Possibly for the first time ever, I'd like you to actually get in touch with what you're really feeling. Don't suppress it. Feel what your body and mind are innately trying to tell you.

The 9 emotional triggers listed below are from the book, *Many Lives Many Masters,* by Brian Weiss.[1] As you read over them, see if any resonate with you. If so, try to begin looking more deeply into why that may be, and what the toxic underlying feeling is that is keeping you stuck there.

In parenthesis, I pose questions that may help you answer and identify the true triggers.

9 TOXIC EMOTIONS
BITTERNESS

Bitterness shows you where you need to heal, where you're still holding judgements on others and yourself. (Who, or what event do you feel bitterness towards? How can you forgive that person or event, if not for them, but for yourself?)

RESENTMENT

Resentment shows you where you're living in the past and not allowing the present to be as it is. (What is it that you resent? How can you turn that around to view it as a learning experience that is leading you to be a more well-rounded, caring individual?)

DISCOMFORT

Discomfort shows you that you need to pay attention right now to what is happening, because you're being given the opportunity to change, to do something different than how you typically do it. (It's important to realize that you will always feel discomfort when taking your life to the next level – this is a protective mechanism in your mind, to keep you safe and stuck in your current "comfort zone," even if it's not a pleasant one. What are your current uncomfortable thoughts or feelings?)

ANGER

Anger shows you what you're passionate about, where your boundaries are, and what you believe needs to change about the world. (Anger can be beneficial if it doesn't burn you out, poison your immune system with increased cortisol, and spill into all areas of your life. Anger must be a temporary emotion channeled into a worthy pursuit or cause. What is your worthy cause you can reframe into something more positive?)

DISAPPOINTMENT

Disappointment shows you that you tried for something, that you do not give in to apathy, that you still are. (Disappointment is a normal human emotion. The issue is that we must move on from it. Learn from each experience and channel that emotion into how you can improve for the next challenge. What can you learn from your disappointments?)

GUILT

Guilt shows you that you're still living in other people's expectations of what you should do (or be). (Parents, friends, religions, schools, work, and other social factors can make you believe you're supposed to fit a specific mold or expectation. Once you allow yourself to be you, and do what you want in life while realizing that you do not owe anyone anything, the guilt will be released. Do you feel any guilt right now?)

SHAME

Shame shows you that you're internalizing other people's beliefs about who you should be (or who you feel you are) and that you need to reconnect with yourself. (This emotion ties in with guilt and shares the same imbalanced mental state. No one can make you feel shame, unless you accept their version of you. When you live a life you can be proud of, and respect yourself, shame will become a non-factor. Do you feel shame around any particular events or around certain people?)

ANXIETY

Anxiety shows you that you need to wake up, right now, and that you need to be present, that you're stuck in the past and living in fear of the future. (Having seen hundreds of people in my practice with anxiety, I can tell you that many people fear what the future may hold, or more specifically not hold for them. Once you change your perspective and give gratitude for what you do have, anxiety ceases to exist. What are your biggest sources of anxiety right now?)

SADNESS

Sadness shows you the depth of your feeling, the depth of your care for others and this world. (While sadness will always be part of the human experience, it's our ability to pull ourselves out of this state that keeps us healthy. When you find yourself sad, feel the feeling – don't deny it. But then, move your mind back to the "now." Use perspective and gratitude for what you do have to help you reach a more positive mental state. Is there a certain issue that makes you sad? If so, can it have a happy ending? If not, how can you still make the best of it, accept it, learn from it, and move forward with your life?)

THE MOST COMMON EMOTIONS

Out of all of the emotional meanings just mentioned, the two most common emotions I see come up on a weekly basis in my practice are anxiety and overwhelm. Literally, a week doesn't go by that I don't hear someone talk about an underlying level of anxiety that is affecting their mood and health.

Those two emotions are ultimately interconnected and, when left unchecked, can fill up your rain barrel and burn out your adrenals through too high of a nor/epinephrine (adrenaline) and cortisol output. If it goes on long enough this can lead to apathy and depression.

YOUR THOUGHTS AFFECT YOUR MOOD

From my experience, it's difficult to get excited about anything when your body and mind are exhausted. I believe a depressed (burned out) body leads a to a depressed mind. As I've mentioned before, there is no separation between mind and body. To heal one, you must heal the other.

Remember, our outward experience of life is largely dictated by our thoughts and our thoughts are absolutely influenced by our mood (This will be explained more in the last chapter) – and part of this issue is that we get locked into a cycle of thinking that seems near impossible to break.

But, like anything that relates to our current health, *there is always an answer.* Before we get to those solutions let's take a self-survey to draw out some of your more limiting, depressing beliefs about yourself.

It is *these limiting beliefs* that are holding you back from smiling more, being more, and having unlimited energy!

Take a moment right now to answer these questions honestly:

WHAT ARE YOUR LIMITING BELIEFS?

- Do you believe you can achieve total health?
- Do you like how your body looks?
- Can you see yourself living in your ideal body?
- Do you believe there is no upper limit to what you can achieve?
- Do you believe you can be truly happy?
- What do you think about most of your day – Are they happy thoughts?
- How do you talk to yourself – Are you kind? Do you build yourself up?
- Do you feel you can achieve the life you've always wanted?

In addition to these questions I would ask how do you picture yourself? Is it usually at your ideal or at your worst?

These are important questions, since the way you think frames what you expect to get out of life. You will always get more of what you think about – your actions will attract those things towards what you constantly think about. So, if you answered "no" multiple times in the questions above, I would urge you to truly work on your mindset for long-term health and well-being in both mind and body.

Beyond the actual answers, I'm also even more interested in you understanding *how you felt* rather than merely what you thought or wrote down when answering the above questions.

Did you feel low energy answering them, or did you begin to light up and feel alive? The answer to that question is all I need to hear to understand where you're at.

REFRAME YOUR VISION

In a moment, I'll share with you some simple at-home Functional Medicine lab tests to run to see if there is an actual bio-chemical imbalance holding you back as well, but for now you must understand that if you feel weak, small, or unmotivated when you view yourself and future, you must correct this.

Unless you begin to dispel any visions you have of yourself as a victim or someone that can't be helped, the odds that you will get better is not good. I only state this because the mind and body are intricately connected and your psychology (thinking) ultimately effects your physiology (body).

This connection is so strong that it's now very easy for me to spot the people that will have the most difficulty in getting well again. They're always the ones that believe they've tried it all and nothing works. They feel that they are destined to live a life of hardship and suffering. They may have seen family members suffer the same fate and they believe there's nothing they can do. They play it off as just poor genetics or another passing excuse that allows them to stay complacent.

I feel for those people and I want so badly to help them, but I know that the first step must come from them in believing they can become well again. This is also a very personal topic for me as well. I was that despondent sick kid who didn't believe he could get well again. I had good reason.

I had been to over 2 dozen of the top doctors and specialists in Boston, only for them to tell me my health ailments were "all in my head." I used to go into those appointments optimistic that *this* was the doctor that would finally figure it out and heal me… Only to leave depressed an hour later.

I struggled like this for many years. Doctor visit after doctor visit, until I gave up completely. I couldn't take anymore reinforcement that *no one was ever* going to figure out how to help me get well. Years went by with no real relief and many relapses along the way.

CREATE YOUR OWN TURNING POINT

Then, one day in my early 20's after another night of not sleeping and lying awake all night, I decided I wasn't going to live this angry, depressed, and unhappy life anymore.

I made a conscious choice from that day on to become the person I wanted to be. I wanted to be happy. I wanted to enjoy life. I wanted to live with more energy and passion. I also wanted to be free of dis-ease and poor health. I didn't know how any of that *was going to happen*, but I was now committed to the process of finding that life for myself.

Did I have relapses in both my attitude and physical symptoms after I made that commitment? Absolutely – But I always made sure I went back to my goal of reshaping my life. I had nothing to lose and after a while, the process actually started to get easier.

By mere *chance*, I met some amazing Naturopaths and health practitioners shortly after my new commitment to heal myself, and they helped me pinpoint where to focus my efforts. Was it coincidence, or was I finally at a point mentally that I was ready to heal physically?

Regardless, I found the answers that had alluded me for so long and the rest is history…

I can honestly say, I don't even resemble the same person I was 15 years ago. My mindset is that of a new person. I love life and I look at it as an amazing adventure. This new thought process allows me to still have the same stress I'd ordinarily have, but my reaction to life's events is completely different.

I now see challenges – not insurmountable obstacles. My energy is better than ever, and today, I can't even believe I used to struggle to mount the stairs to my bedroom, or that I would be too tired to even talk to other people!

My life has changed and it all started with recognizing my limiting beliefs, dominant thoughts, and then controlling my emotions. At the time, I didn't know my rain barrel was so full of stress, fear and negativity. Now I do. This is what I want for you to realize as well. I do not have any special abilities' and I certainly wasn't taught this growing up or in schools. Almost no one is.

IT'S TIME TO GET FED UP

So how did I change my mindset?

What happened was that I got fed up. I couldn't live with the emotions I was struggling with. I felt like a victim. I felt helpless. I felt weak. These are all qualities I didn't want for myself.

So, I want to ask you just like I've asked thousands of others before you – What do you want for your life? How do you want to feel? How do you want to see yourself? What fires you up and gives you energy?

Don't answer what you think you should be saying, but instead shoot for your ideal. *Don't place any limits on yourself.* Journal and speak out loud, "What does your best-self and ideal life look and feel like?"

You must first get very clear on *what you want for you.* (Note: never focus on what you do not want since you are then still inadvertently focusing on it.) It's only after you have this clarity can you begin to take the proper steps to achieve it. Everything begins with thought – our emotions then form from there. All of the great masters have shared this philosophy since the beginning of time…

After you get clear on how you would like to live your life, begin to become aware of your thoughts from moment to moment. You may find they are more limiting and negative than you'd like. Don't try to fight them. Arguing against anything only gives it more life. Instead, simply and quickly shift your mind to a new positive thought – one that serves you. Go back to focusing on what you do want.

In time, this flipping of thoughts will become more natural. You'll also have to do it less as your subconscious becomes reprogrammed with the new idea you have for yourself and your life. Although this process may seem somewhat metaphysical or esoteric I can assure you it is not.

THE SCIENCE OF EMOTIONS

Quantum physics and medical science have validated these exact sentiments and even have a name for the part of the brain that draws your goals closer to you. It's called the Reticular Activating System (RAS).

Its job is to filter out the millions of data points you see all around you at every second and only make you aware of what serves you the most. Keep in mind, this isn't always positive, since your dominant thoughts allow your mind to see what data points it seeks. It is literally a self-fulfilling prophecy, which is why you'll get more of what you think about the most.

At the risk of sounding too "out there," I simply want to say that letting go of your current emotional make-up is oftentimes the ultimate hurdle to truly getting well, losing the weight, and living the life you've always wanted.

In terms of emptying your rain barrel, understanding and owning your emotions is just as important as any of the individual DESTRESS Protocols™ you've already read about. It holds the key to lasting results and a snowball effect of getting more of what you do want in life.

So before we move on to the actual bio-chemical imbalances that may be keeping you feeling "stuck," I'd like to share with you 7 tips for beginning to re-create your new emotional-state:

HOW TO CHANGE YOUR EMOTIONS
START WITH AWARENESS

The only way to begin to get control of your life, is to first become aware of your thoughts.

Now, I know this may seem obvious, but I can assure you most people jump from emotion to emotion without truly stepping back to see what programming is running through their mind.

The best way to do this is to become a 3rd party bystander that is simply listening to the thoughts that are running through your head. What are they saying to you? Is it negative? Are they holding you down or back from achieving what you want out of life? Do they serve you in any positive way?

Simply take notes on what you are thinking throughout the day and in specific situations.

This practice is the cornerstone to being able to eventually disassociate yourself from the "monkey mind" we all have that is continually playing on a loop the childhood and accumulated lifetime of information that is meant to protect us from dangers. It serves its purpose, but not without potential harm as well. Once you realize that it is not you, but instead the accumulated data sending messages from your subconscious in response to every situation you find yourself in, then you can begin to reprogram that data.

BREATHE AND RELAX

I mentioned breathing a few times now throughout this book. There's a reason for that. You will probably never find a supplement, nootropic, medication, or technique more profound than returning to your breath.

Once you begin to focus back on your breathing, you'll notice that most of the time when you're stressed or feeling anxious you're most likely not breathing. You're probably holding your breath. And when you do take a breath it's just shallow chest breaths. Your goal should be to slow your breathing and begin to take deeper more relaxed belly breaths.

By just taking 3-5 slow deep belly breaths (ideally eyes closed) and really focusing on feeling the air come in through your nose and into your lungs for a count of about 5 seconds and then feel toxic air being expelled through your mouth over a slower 7 second count, I have no doubt the negative emotions will begin to pass.

One of the reasons this works so well is that it is challenging for your mind to hold its focus on two tasks at once. By returning to your breathing you will effectively cancel out the stressor. And, by slowly releasing your breath, while at the same time bringing more oxygen into your body, you will activate the parasympathetic nervous system, which is naturally calming.

(For more information on belly breathing check out StephenCabral.com/podcasts)

Once you become aware of stressful situations, you will ultimately find that you can use this calming breath technique to defuse your response to what your mind deems a fight or flight situation. In time, you will also find your personal triggers and eliminate situations you used to find stressful. This will also help you lower the cortisol response and as a result lose weight and feel better.

PRACTICE NON-JUDGEMENT

I grew up judging everything. I viewed myself and everything I did as either better than or worse than the object of my judgement. Eventually, I learned that this led to a cause of my anxiety and burn out. I felt life was a competition.

And worse, on a subconscious level, if you're always passing judgement, you always believe that you yourself are being judged. This is a secret few have been made aware of. For me, it was a life-changing switch. I stopped judging, so judgement was no longer on my mind. Therefore, I no longer thought anyone was judging me. I was now free to be me.

From now on as you begin to compare yourself or judge another person, simply catch yourself, take a deep breath, and smile as you let it pass…

UNDERSTANDING STRESS

It's all of our jobs to understand that stress is something we perceive. It reality it doesn't exist.

To prove this, you simply have to look at varying levels of stress allocated to any given situation depending on the person. For example, some people love public speaking, others believe that it's a fate worse than death.

"Stress" is an outward symptom of an alleged threat of some type to our well-being. Although this served us well thousands of years ago, most of us are no longer in danger of famine, the weather, or being eaten by another animal. Although I won't deny some situations seem to be more universally stressful, we do always have a choice. We get to respond how we'd like.

I'm not perfect, and I'm not expecting you to be either. My recommendation is to feel the stress for a moment, understand why you had that emotion, and then let it pass just as it came. Go back to your breath and let it go as best and quickly as you can. Better things lie ahead…

BEGIN WITH YOUR MIND

Many people believe that they're just one magic pill or potion away from being well again. And while nutritional supplements can often make all the difference in the world, they still aren't stronger than your own mind. (More on this to come in the last chapter.)

So, if you're hopping from doctor to doctor, my recommendation is not to seek further help until you work on you first. You must first come to the uncomfortable conclusion that it may just be you that is holding you back.

The tricky part is that your subconscious emotions, previous programming, and self-limiting thoughts may be telling your body a different story than the one you consciously recite. You may be actively saying you want to get well, lose the weight, and feel great, but at a deeper level, that may not be the case.

Unfortunately, I've seen many people continue to play the role of the victim due to misinterpreted spiritual aspirations, or the sympathy they get from others due to their condition.

The way to find out if you're secretly sabotaging your results is to see if your actions match up to your conscious desires. Are you taking care of yourself, eating the right foods, exercising, getting to bed on time, or working to improve your mindset? If not, start here. This tip will save you years of struggle and thousands of dollars in doctor's visits before you're ready to make permanent change in your life.

THE DAILY MANTRA

About a century ago, Emile Coue, a French psychologist, came up with a mantra to help his patients get well. (A mantra is simply a saying you recite to yourself over and over that brings meaning and sinks deep into your subconscious the more your repeat it.)

Emile Coue had his patients repeat, *"Every day in every way, I am getting better."*

That's it – Just that one line.

It's so simple, but yet powerful enough for his patients to credit this mantra with helping them to overcome issues they had struggled with for years.

Is it the placebo effect at work here? Absolutely. But since when is that a bad thing? The placebo effect often beats medication in head to head clinical trials against some of the "top drugs." It also goes to show that your own body and mind can manufacture what it needs based on your thoughts and feelings.

For your own mantra, you can use Coue's, or you can replace the word, "better," with a goal of yours. However, my recommendation is to keep the mantra as stated above, since "better" is more general and will allow for many areas in your life to improve.

This simple technique is best recited when you first wake up, when you're looking in the mirror, and before bed. Try to recite it multiple times in a row and really *feel yourself feeling better*. You have nothing to lose, and everything to gain!

PERFECTION IS NEVER THE END GOAL

As I explained earlier in this chapter, the mere thought of having to be perfect or control every one of your thoughts is yet another cause of stress.

Once you realize perfection is unattainable, you can then aim for a modified version of it as a goal, with the understanding that you're simply going to do your best. Some days will be easier than others. That's part of life.

My goal, is to have you be gentler on yourself and recognize that simply moving in the right direction each day is a win. The reason this is so powerful, is due to the fact that if you keep moving in the direction of your goal you will eventually achieve it.

The timeline is irrelevant.

Once you put demands on when you must achieve the perfect health, body, life, happiness, etc., you're once again filling up your rain barrel with stress, expectations, and future-casted judgment of whether you lived up to expectations.

Be kind to yourself. You're doing the best you can, given your current situation and programming. You'll do better in time and you will continue to grow. Continual growth is the real goal – not perfection.

IT GETS EASIER

I remember when I first took up skiing. I started a little later in life and all I can remember is that I used to cross the tips of my skis every time I got worried about falling. Of course, if you've ever skied you know crossing your skis is a recipe for falling face first into the snow!

Eventually, I learned to control the distance of my skis from each other as well as some of the advanced techniques of staying on the "edges." The amazing thing was that once I put in the practice, and got to the advanced stages of skiing, never once did I have to think about not crossing the tips of my skis – It came naturally.

Remember, for most of us, whenever we try anything new we falter the first few times (or 50 times!). It's normal to fall down at first… We need to understand this. Being hard on yourself is simply a bad habit that can broken when you become aware you're doing it.

Failure is just an opportunity to learn more about yourself and the world. In fact, most things I've failed at have become my talents and assets because I worked so hard to overcome my failings that as a side effect, I became a master of that art, hobby, sport, etc.

In time, working on your breathing, releasing negative emotions, and envisioning a greater healthier future for yourself will be all you know. Work harder on yourself than you do on anything else – after that everything else you want in life will fall into place.

CHEMICAL IMBALANCES

My love for studying psychology is only surpassed by that of digging deep into the science of bioregulatory medicine and biochemical responses due to our environment.

This has led to some amazing discoveries that I've been able to incorporate into my practice on how our psychological state can often be a byproduct of our physiological terrain. In normal speak, that essentially means that our mind is affected by what's going on in our body.

Now that we've reviewed some of the more important aspects on working on your psychology, let's look at the other half of the equation.

(Note: Even after reading about the biochemical imbalances below, you absolutely should not disregard everything in this chapter that was already stated. Using the techniques from above will only help you heal faster and potentiate the effects of any additional nutritional compounds.)

Sometimes, our emotions are harder to control than we'd like. It seems as if no matter what you do, it's not enough. You may feel like a dark cloud is following you around, or that you can't shake your anxiousness, or irritability. When these feelings become a chronic fixture in your life it's time to go deeper.

But, before we get to which lab tests and supplements I recommend in order to rebalance your body, let's first talk about why you may be feeling overwhelmed, anxious, depressed, or stressed from a physiological (bodily) perspective.

One unexpected consequence of working with thousands of people on their health is that I've had the privilege of understanding how much the state of the body effects the brain. Previously, I shared how your brain affects your body, but your body is just as capable of sending feedback to your brain.

And if the feedback is that of pain, suffering, inflammation, or injury, your mind sends you those same signals (as thoughts and feelings) that something is wrong.

A 2-SIDED APPROACH

This is why although I whole heartedly recommend therapy or counseling (that focuses on healing – not reliving the pain), I know that in most cases people need to correct their physiology. Without this partnership, the results of therapy are often poor, which is why so many people remain in counseling for years…

But where do you look in your body for what is imbalanced so that you can finally get your emotional and mental health back in balance? That is the ultimate question, and it's one that has both an easy *and* a complex answer.

The easy answer is to look directly at the part of the body that ails you the most. Do you have bloating, headaches, insomnia, poor energy, skin issues, weight gain, or an auto-immune disease? Think about this really hard for a moment, because the answers I share with you below could finally heal years of pain.

DIGESTION

If you're unsure of where to start begin with your digestion. As I stated earlier, your "feel good, happy neurotransmitter" called serotonin is produced mainly in your intestines. Literally, 90% of all of serotonin is made in your gut.[2] Therefore, if your digestive tract is inflamed or imbalanced you may have a difficult time being "happy."

From a clinical perspective, when something is wrong with your digestion you may not actually be able to produce the happy, calming neurotransmitters you need to battle depression, anxiety, obsessive compulsive disorder, and more. A simple at-home urine test called the Organic Acids Test, can help you look to see if you have candida, bacterial overgrowth, or other issues with your gut. If you suspect a h. pylori or a parasite, you may opt instead for a stool test.

CORTISOL

Too much of the stress hormone cortisol can make you feel irritable, anxious, high-strung, and on edge. It can also lead to poor sleep and insomnia. Too little cortisol can make you feel depressed, lethargic, and apathetic. Testing a 24-hour saliva adrenal cortisol test right at home, can help you determine if you have balanced levels of or not.

ESTROGEN

Both men and women can struggle with estrogen dominance. As explained earlier, this is often due to a lowered availability of progesterone. Why?

Because when we get stressed, our bodies need to make more cortisol fast, and in absence of ready cortisol, we turn to the *precursor for cortisol*, instead, which is progesterone. This is where we get a progesterone lack and estrogen excess.

Although women (and men) can have completely normal levels of estrogen on a lab test, they get all of the irritability, bloating, skin issues, and depression/mood issues that come along with estrogen dominance due to their low levels of progesterone.

The same saliva cortisol (adrenal) hormone lab mentioned above tests estrogen and progesterone (as well as DHEA and testosterone).

LOW AMBITION & DRIVE

Although many factors can zap your zest for life and ambition, low hormones like DHEA and testosterone can be a cause. Libido, confidence, and all those alpha qualities typically go hand in hand with adequate hormone levels of both of these hormones.

Unfortunately, due to age, stress, poor nutrition, lack of exercise, and actual biological aging factors can all result in a decline in DHEA and testosterone. The great news is that there are safe, non-hormone replacement therapies that boost your own natural levels.

To see if you could use a boost, you can use that same hormone saliva lab mentioned above. This one lab gives you the results of all your hormone levels. This is an important note, since dysregulated cortisol is often times at the center for low sex hormones.

So, if you want to rebalance your anti-aging, feel good hormones you must decrease stress and cortisol output. As a side benefit, lower levels of cortisol may help stave off Alzheimer's and dementia.[3]

FOOD SENSITIVITIES

One of the most overlooked causes of depression, anxiety, obsessive compulsive disorder, panic attacks, and other mental health issues, is hidden food sensitivities.

It's still astonishing to me how children and adults that eliminate the foods they find are sensitivities to them from an IgG or other food sensitivity test, can literally turn their life around.

It really can be that powerful. The reason is simple. If you're sensitive to a food and you eat it, you are causing an inflammatory reaction in your body. This inflammation doesn't just stay in your gut. It effects your entire body and brain.[4]

My recommendation is to begin by eliminating the foods listed in the Diet section of the DESTRESS Protocol™, or following Dr. Cabral

Detox program outlined in this book's last section. If you want more personalized recommendations, you can run an at-home food sensitivity test.

INFLAMMATION

Inflammation can come in many forms. Some of them are from all the environmental toxins that we spoke about in Part 1, others come from the foods we eat, and then of course there's stress.

However, one issue I see over and over again in my Functional Medicine practice is the alarming rate of Omega-6 to Omega-3 levels in people's blood. Keep in mind that Omega-6 fats are more inflammatory. We need them, and they do serve an important purpose, but we just don't want them to overpower our anti-inflammatory fats, which are our Omega-3s.

The average American has a ratio of about 16:1 in terms of Omega-6 to Omega-3s in their blood.[5] The ideal ratio is closer to 2 or 3:1 maximum. Now can you start to see why both our brain and body may be so inflamed?

To decrease your Omega-6 fats, try to cut back on processed grains, vegetable oils, and conventionally farmed meat, eggs, and milk. To increase your omega-3 levels, include more vegetables, wild fish, walnuts, flax, chia seeds, and sea vegetables.

To find out your Omega 6 to Omega 3 ratio and to see to what degree inflammation may be affecting you, you can run an at-home blood spot card lab test.

(Note: All lab tests mentioned in this book can be requested by your Functional Medicine Doctor or found at StephenCabral.com/rbe on the resource page to run yourself right in the privacy of your own home.)

ADD/ADHD

There are so many labels placed on children and adults now that I can't list every one. So, whether your child (or you) has been told you have ADD, ADHD, executive function disorder, or another medical term for a group of symptoms it's time to look deeper.

High levels of copper, or heavy metals like mercury and aluminum can damage the nervous system and brain.

Plus, low levels of magnesium deficiency can be a simple cause for having difficulty calming down. Additionally, poor blood sugar regulation (hypoglycemia) can be a deeper underlying root cause of stress, anxiety, irritability, headaches, or difficulty concentrating.

To test for these levels, I highly recommend looking at a Hair Tissue Mineral Analysis. This lab will provide you with every mineral data point you need to recognize your mineral deficiencies and heavy metal toxicities.

Please also keep in mind that learning difficulties and behavioral outbursts have been tied to increased intestinal permeability (leaky gut), food dyes (red, yellow & blue food "coloring."), as well as food sensitivities.

My recommendation is to run both a Hair Tissue Mineral Analysis and an Organic Acids Test for the confirmation of hidden toxicities if you or a child suffers from any mood or learning based issue.

GENETICS

I for one will never allow anyone to use the excuse that they have "bad genes…"

I did this personally for years, but blaming your genes for your mental or physical health is just a way to shirk your responsibility for your own health. –

It's almost like using the genetics excuse to justify why you aren't willing to take the first step to getting well.

Again, I say this because I am someone with multiple genetic mutations that allow for the expression of unhealthy inflammation, high stress hormone output, and poor detoxification, *if* I don't control my lifestyle and environment.

Having said that, genetics do play a role in our emotional well-being. Those of us with methylation issues have trouble keeping inflammation down and as result must be more careful with how we eat and take certain supplements (like methylated b-vitamins) to stay more balanced.

Some people (myself included) also have a presupposition towards higher adrenal output (MR genotype/snp), which can lead to increased irritability, anger, rage, etc.

It can also lead to burn out, due to a decreased ability to calm yourself down. However, once you know this you can begin to modify your lifestyle and use calming herbal adaptogens and minerals to keep you balanced.

In my practice, I work with the top genetic lab in the world to test both online and Boston wellness clients for all these issues. The lab results come with an impressive 97-page personal DNA report.

(Note: For a full scope of the at-home labs I recommend please see the resources page for this book. I have no affiliation with any labs and if a better lab becomes available I will list it as part of my top lab recommendations. You may run these labs with your own doctor or through us at StephenCabral.com/rbe)

SUPPLEMENTS

For the most part, I do not buy into all of these new mood-altering nootropic supplements.

The reason for this is that they are created by so-called "biohackers" that have never studied the real cause behind a low neurotransmitter issue or other factors leading to a poor mental outlook. As a result, they add a dash of this and splash of that without full regard as to what these compounds can do – and when mixed together.

However, what I can recommend (if you decide not to go the testing route) is to stay with safe, tried and true formulas made by Functional Medicine companies such as Pure Ecologics, Thorne, Integrative Therapeutics, Orthomolecular Medicine, and Equilibrium Nutrition.

Here are a list of beneficial supplements that can potentially improve your mood and help you reshape your emotions as you begin to Empty Your Rain Barrel™ of toxic thoughts that are holding you back.

BENEFICIAL BOTANICALS

- Ashwagandha
- Passionflower
- Lemonbalm
- Chamomile
- Rhodiola (for balanced energy)
- Valerian Root
- Kava Kava
- Maca
- CBD oil (this is not marijuana and contains little to no THC)

All of the earth-grown herbs listed above can act as natural sedatives and help to down regulate high cortisol and stress.

Many also act as adaptogens, so if you're feeling too low, they give you a boost in both mental and physical energy, and if you're getting too stressed they help calm you down. My personal favorites are ashwgandha and rhodiola for calming daytime stress, while at the same time boosting energy.

NEUROTRANSMITTERS & HORMONES

- **GABA**
  (Natural anti-anxiety)
- **5-HTP**
  (Precursor to serotonin. Do not take with SSRIs)
- **l-Tyrosine**
  (Can improve focus, energy, and thyroid)
- **Phosphatidyl Serine**
  (Calms high cortisol levels as found on adrenal lab test)
- **Melatonin**
  (Aids in sleep. Typically only needed for short-term use.)

I typically reserve neurotransmitter balancing hormones for acute cases that involve extreme health imbalances. I also only use them in the short-term, and very rarely would I use them initially, since supplementing with them does not treat a root cause issue. After about 12-16 weeks, I will begin to slowly wean someone off of them.

VITAMINS

- **Methyl B12**
  (Methylcobalamin or adenosylcobalamin)
- **Methyl Folate**
  (NatureFolate™ or 5-MTHF)
- **B6**
  (pyridoxine 5 phosphate)

- **B-Vitamin Complex**
  (Contains the entire b-vitamin family)
- **Vitamin C**

I always opt for the methylated form of B-12 and folic acid. The reason for this is that about 1/3 of the population has genetic variances in their DNA that does not allow them to fully utilize those two vitamins.

This means that the synthetic versions such as cyanocobalamin and folic acid cannot fully be utilized and, at the worst, can actually build up in your system and become toxic. For just a few dollars more, I'd choose the Functional Medicine absorbable form.

I also find b-vitamins work better when used as one synergistic formula. I usually start most people at around ½-1 serving of a b-complex vitamin with breakfast. Then if needed, I will add additional B-12, B6, methyl folate, etc. Since most high quality Functional Medicine multi-vitamins or all-in-one shakes contain a b-vitamin complex already, additional b-complex supplementation may not ever be needed.

MINERALS

- Calcium
- Magnesium
- Sodium
- Potassium
- Iodine
- Chromium
- Selenium
- Zinc

There are many minerals you could be taking, but in order for your cardiovascular and nervous system to function properly all your electrolytes like calcium, magnesium, sodium, and potassium need to be balanced and at adequate levels (as seen on a HTMA/hair test). Too much or too little will lead to anxiety, stress burn out, and apathy. A lot of the time, the ratio, rather than the total amount can be *more important* in keeping the body stable and balanced.

Also, proper energy and metabolism rely on having enough iodine and selenium reserves to fully maximize thyroid hormone.

As an aside, chromium is vital to regulating blood sugar levels and ensuring you don't get irritable, aggressive, or fatigued. And finally, zinc can be a tremendous anabolic mineral used to rebuild every tissue in your body, as well as boost beneficial fat-burning, muscle building, and anti-aging hormones.

IT'S TIME TO TURN YOUR LIFE AROUND

No one said transforming your body and mind was supposed to be easy – But it's absolutely worth it!

Although I love watching people heal from years of physical health struggles, my favorite part is watching their emotional life turn around. I enjoy seeing how their thought process has been upgraded as well.

Truthfully, it's difficult to become fully well again without improving all aspects of your mental and physical life. I've literally seen the worst of the worst get well again and leave the apathy, fatigue, brain fog, anxiety, depression, and learning difficulties behind them. And if they can do it, I have no doubt you can *and will* as well…

We're approaching the final pieces of the DESTRESS Protocol™, and this next chapter distills 20 years of repairing and rebalancing your body into one easy to digest plan. I can't wait to share with you how you can combine the best of ancient healing secrets with state-of-the-art Functional Medicine!

EMPTY YOUR RAIN BARREL™ STARTING WITH AWARENESS

You've learned a lot in this chapter. So much so, that I may even recommend a 2nd read if you feel it could help reinforce certain ideas and concepts.

And, if you're looking for just one place to begin, I can't recommend enough this one starting point – It is to become more aware of what you think, feel, and experience throughout the day.

Become an outside observer of your own inner thoughts. Do not judge them. Simply listen to your mind and see what it is saying and thinking. Many people have never done this. It is really key to helping to see how your own thinking may have become toxic and how it might be destroying your life by filling up your rain barrel on a daily basis.

You can do this with just about all your negative, toxic thoughts about yourself and others. Are the majority of your thoughts negative, sad, shameful, or are they positive, uplifting and happy? If they're mixed, then what events or situations cause them to change?

At this point in your health journey, you just want to start seeing correlations and becoming aware of your most prevalent thoughts. It is these thoughts that eventually lead to actions, which become your habits and routines, that ultimately become your life. When you start to become aware of your thoughts, then you can begin to reprogram those thoughts with more positive ones. Of course, this will take some time and patience, but if you're willing to work this process amazing things will begin to transpire in your life.

Becoming aware is the starting point to your entire transformation and the new life that awaits you…

Supplements

If you're like me and those in my Functional Medicine practice, you probably want to get well or lose the excess weight as fast as possible.

You're not looking to take the long, winding road to getting well or getting your "mojo" back...

The trick is discovering how to do this without sacrificing long-term health for faster results. The answer to this lies in time-tested and scientifically proven nutritional supplements.

COMMON MISCONCEPTIONS

Some people don't like the idea of taking nutritional supplements, but often, that's because they don't understand what is really in their supplements. Often, you don't even know what is in OTC vitamins and supplements, especially those sold on the internet. Indeed, you just might be buying baking soda in a capsule...

But high quality Functional Medicine supplements – typically—are organic, harvested from reliable sources and are things your body really needs to be in perfect harmony, balance, and health.

Typically, functional health supplements are concentrates of vitamins, minerals, herbs, whole foods, and other natural products meant to speed up the healing process. These nutritional supplements provide what your body is lacking, or help to remove what you have too much of (toxins).

Remember, you do not have an endless storehouse of vitamins and nutrients that your body can draw from. Your reserves can get so low in certain minerals, trace minerals, vitamins, and fatty acids that you actually begin to break down your own muscle tissue, organs, and demineralize your bone in order to maintain equilibrium. *(One of the best example of this is osteoporosis, in which the body leaches calcium and other minerals from your bones.)*

This is certainly not what we want – But no one gets an adequate supply of the many nutrients we very much need on a daily basis.[1]

What's even worse, according to the *Centers for Disease Control and Prevention*, in 2012 more than one-third of children and adolescents aged 6 to 19 are considered overweight or obese.[2] However, even though these children are overweight they also are lacking in basic nutrients. Greater than 90% of children from age 4 to 18 don't meet the current recommendations for vegetable intake, and more than 75% don't meet guidelines for healthy fruit intake.[3]

Even if you believe you eat an incredibly healthy diet, it's still likely you do not meet your daily vitamin & mineral requirements. Here's why:

WHERE DID THE NUTRIENTS GO? DEPLETED SOIL

By now, you've probably read that although conventionally grown and organic foods both have the same exact *macro*nutrient profile, their *micro*nutrient profiles vary greatly. Organic fruits and vegetables *do* contain more vitamins, minerals, and phytonutrients.[4]

However, due to soil depletion, even organic food still doesn't contain the same nutrient profile it did just 60 years ago. Because of this, we aren't getting as much nutrition out of our food. From 1950 – 1999, the infamous

Donald Davis study published in the *Journal of the American College of Nutrition* found these decreases in fruits & vegetables:

- 6% less protein
- 16% less calcium
- 9% less phosphorus
- 15% less iron
- 38% less riboflavin (B2)
- 20% less vitamin C[5]

MATURITY AT HARVEST

Unfortunately, the statistics above come from fruit and vegetables picked when they fully ripen. However, many foods you're purchasing at grocery stores are picked before the produce is ripe so that it will not be rotten by the time it makes it to your local shopping center.

Picking fruit and vegetables before they're ripe leads to a further decrease in vitamins, minerals, and antioxidants. For example, picking a tomato and storing it for 5 days before it is eaten decreases vitamin C by another 13%.[6]

HIGH CARBON ATMOSPHERE

Since the quality of the air we breathe is also needed by the plants we're trying to grow, they are affected just the same exact way. However, in the case of growing food, it's been found that the increased CO_2 in the atmosphere from pollution is decreasing important minerals and compounds such as nitrogen, potassium, magnesium, and protein.[7]

LOW-CALORIE DIETS

While low calorie diets may help you lose weight in the short-term, the longer lasting effects can be a gradual depletion of your own vital reserves. The reason for this is that you simply can't get enough of the vitamins, minerals, and other nutrients needed for proper anti-aging and health.

CHEAP FERTILIZERS

Most big farming corporations only care about large yields and lowering costs. Therefore, when it comes to choosing a fertilizer they opt for the lowest cost item to get the job done. This is why nitrogen fertilizers with added phosphorus and potassium have become so popular.

However, when these isolated nutrients are added at the expense of a full-spectrum of minerals, plants do not get the full nutritional benefits from them. This means, the plants are created with lower levels of minerals – especially calcium and magnesium which are reduced with potassium fertilizers.[8]

SKIPPING BREAKFAST

Skipping breakfast can be helpful for some, but if you are active, or have a job (school) that requires increased cognitive ability or manual labor, it can be quite harmful.[9,10]

Eating breakfast can leave your body scrambling to catch up for calories and nutrition later in the day – trying to squeeze it into just 1 or 2 meals. For many individuals, skipping breakfast also leads to a desire for sugar or processed foods, which are devoid of the nutrients your body needs to be healthy.

Lastly, for some body types like the ectomorph (Vata) passing on breakfast can lead to an increased catabolic environment within their body, which means they may suffer muscle loss, hypoglycemia, mood disturbance (anxiety, irritability, overwhelm), and fatigue.

GRAIN-FED MEAT

It's literally a travesty what we've turned our farming practices into in the United States…

Cows are now being fed genetically modified (GMO) corn, soy, and other foods that they were never meant to eat. They're even given truckloads of Skittles candy to fatten them up faster.[11]

And since the food they're given and the horrible, bacteria and virus-ridden conditions they are raised in makes them sick, they are then prophylactically given antibiotics to keep them alive. We're now at the point that more than 60% of all the antibiotics in the US are given to animals – not humans.[12]

In turn, this horrific practice leads to a fattening up of the cows, chickens, and other animals, as well as to general malnourishment of the actual animal – which is eventually sold to consumers as meat.

The same goes for dairy milk and cheese, which is loaded with bacteria, toxins, and often times pus from the diseased cows. Unless, you're choosing free range, grass-fed/finished or pastured meat, you are most likely doing more harm than good for your body.

FARM-RAISED FISH

It's important to understand that farm raised fish of all species can spell disaster for your health in a number of ways.

First, fish were never meant to eat corn, grains, or poultry and pork for that matter. Pollutants found in the fish feed include dioxins, PCBs, and a number of different drugs and chemicals. The type of contaminants that have been detected in farmed salmon have a negative effect on brain development and is associated with autism, ADD/ADHD and reduced IQ.[13]

We also know that these chemicals can affect other organ systems in the body's immune system and metabolism. Farm-raised salmon contain PCBs at a concentration *16 times higher* than wild salmon, and the level of dioxin is also higher, by a factor of 11 – Both of which are cancer-causing chemicals.

Additionally, farmed salmon provides your body with higher levels of inflammation producing omega-6 fatty acids. Inflammation has been linked to almost every disease including cancer, diabetes, arthritis, coronary artery disease, high blood pressure, and even Alzheimer's.

And last, but certainly not least, did you know that farmed salmon are fed pellets of chicken feces, arsenic containing corn meal feed made of grains that were sprayed with tons of pesticides to protect the crops, soy, genetically modified canola oil and other high concentrations of toxins?

My recommendation is to stay clear of this dis-ease causing fish.[14]

AGING & DIGESTION

Now that we know many of the foods we eat don't contain the nutrients they once did, it's important to understand that our digestion also changes as we age.

As we get older, our body's ability to produce hydrochloric acid (HCL) in our stomach goes down. This is called, hypochlorhydria, and it decreases our digestive strength and capability of breaking down protein.

Eventually, this lack of HCL leads to less absorption of crucial nutrients your body needs to stay strong, energetic, metabolically-charged, and aging well. Some of these include a malabsorption of vitamin B12, folate, calcium, magnesium, iron, zinc and trace minerals.

(Note: Acid blocking medications can also cause the same issues stated above, regardless of age.)

A LACK OF FRUITS & VEGETABLES

Since there's been a lot of media hype lately talking about how fruit can make you fat and that you should stay clear of it, we're now suffering the consequences…

Low-glycemic fruit, such as berries, can be beneficial no matter what your health or body transformation goals. Since berries are mainly skin you are getting plenty of fiber to slow the blood sugar response, and the skin contains much of the vitamins, minerals, and phytonutrients your body needs to stay well and combat aging.

As far as vegetables go, the issue I see is that most people never vary their selection. They eat the same 5-6 "go-to" vegetables without ever branching out and *eating a rainbow* of nutrition on their plate.

WATER

The last item I wanted to touch on is the fact that most of us do not have access to pure spring water.

This means the water we're drinking has been filtered of the structure and high mineral content you would find from a stream that has been running over rocks and through the soil. Because of this, the water we now drink lacks the natural calcium, magnesium, sodium, potassium and other trace minerals our body uses to function optimally.

LIVING IN THE MODERN WORLD

Although I try to remain an idealist, I do have to live in the real world.

Because of that, I understand that there has to be some give and take as a trade-off for the conveniences we have in this modern world. It's because of these trade-offs that we must look to nutritional supplements to pick up where our diet leaves off.

One thought worth repeating is that the word "supplement" literally means, "something that completes or enhances something else when added to it."

Therefore, when talking about using nutritional supplements as part of your daily routine, all we're talking about is adding in what you're currently missing – nothing more need be added.

I also prefer to look at supplements as a "fail-safe" to ensure you are not lacking the proper nutrients needed to keep you healthy and balanced. Plus, adding in something as simple as an all-in-one shake or multi-vitamin, and a greens powder can help to detoxify the environmental chemicals you're exposed to on a daily basis.

And, as I explained earlier in the "Toxins" chapter, certain nutrients like b-vitamins, vitamin c, glutamine, and sulfur-based amino acids are crucial in helping your liver to clean your blood and prevent you from accumulating these disease and cancer causing chemicals in your adipose tissue (fat stores) and brain.

Plus, in a Harvard University Physicians long-term study, men were found to decrease their chance for cancer by 8% by simply taking a multi-vitamin each day.[15]

This is just one of thousands of research studies showing the efficacy of using high-quality nutritional supplements to live a healthier and longer life.

WHY HAS THIS BEEN KEPT FROM US?

Although the importance of nutritional supplements has been scientifically proven to help a wide variety of ailments and combat aging, it's still not widely accepted in conventional medicine. This is sad, but it's the world we live in.

The truth is that unless pharmaceutical companies can patent a vitamin, extract, or nutrient, your doctor will most likely never recommend one.

(Note: Germany and other countries are now training many of their physicians in Functional Medicine and nutritional supplement use.)

The problem is that medical school does not provide a foundation for true health. And, only a fraction of medical schools provide even a single nutrition class for graduating doctors!

It's no wonder medical doctors can't speak knowledgably about nutrition or supplementation unless they've gone on to do post-doctoral work after graduation.

In my opinion, the current system of medical school is not actually preparing doctors for helping people get and stay well. "Modern medicine" has actually turned into a form of "sick care" where anyone that suffers from a set of symptoms is given a name of a disease and then medicated for the rest of their life.

This is not healthcare – it's sick care, and it's unfortunate that it is the only form of medicine most people know about.

Because of this, not enough people are exposed to natural health, and if they are, they're often apprehensive since it is not the customary route of medicine in the world.

It's too bad, but when I was studying in India I was told that less than 5% of the country still used Ayurvedic Medicine, which at one time was the oldest and longest standing form of medicine in the world – originating in India. (Once Britain took over India they replaced it with the same style of conventional allopathic medicine practiced in the US and abroad.)

QUALITY OF CARE

There are other differences to be taken in to account though as well…

When you meet with a natural health practitioner your initial appointment is typically 60-90 minutes and your follow-ups are 30-60 minutes long. Contrast that with the 15-minutes you get with your MD and you'll see why that even if your MD could talk with you about healthy lifestyle factors and quality nutritional supplements there's just not time to do so.

Please don't get me wrong, I do appreciate conventional medicine. I absolutely do, and I'm in awe of all the technological break-throughs in surgery and other life-saving acute forms of medicine. My personal belief is that if you have a life-threatening condition you should see a Medical Doctor. However, if you have a chronic condition you must look for the underlying root cause – If you don't you'll only be masking the symptoms with drugs.

I believe in an ideal world, everyone would have both a Primary Care Medical Doctor and Naturopathic Doctor/Functional Medicine Practitioner. This would combine the best of both worlds. What an amazing state of medicine that would be…

So now that we know the goal of the conventional medical system is not to teach you about healthy lifestyle factors such as nutrition, exercise, and supplements, we understand it is up to us to take care of our own bodies.

Hopefully, by now you can see that high quality nutritional supplements should be on that self-care list.

WHAT THE TOP DOCTORS RECOMMEND

In 2016, one of the largest Functional Medicine supplement dispensary shared the results from what the top natural health doctors in medicine were recommending to their patients. [16]

(I'll be sharing those results in just a moment.)

I found this data extremely interesting since it is quite revealing when it comes to what most (natural health) doctors believe will help the greatest amount of people based on the research.

Plus, it's backed up by in-office patient appointments where the doctors get to see if the supplements are actually helping in the real world.

The answer is crystal clear.

Nutritional supplements can save lives. And when you contrast this with the fact that pharmaceutical drugs are the 3rd leading cause of death, you can understand why more and more doctors are trying to minimize the amount of drugs prescribed to everyone.

The problem is, and what I always share in my practice, is that *you can't just do nothing*. Meaning, if you have high blood pressure or cholesterol you can't just say you don't want to take any pharmaceutical drugs because they're dangerous if you don't intend to heal your body naturally – Doing that would leave you potentially susceptible to an early death.

The alternative (technically, there is no alternative) would be to instead look for the root cause through Functional Medicine testing and then implement the information you are reading in this book, as well as a tailored supplement protocol (if needed after doing a full detox and diet).

The bottom line is that as long as you're purchasing your supplements from a reputable online retailer or from a Functional Medicine practice you will be well on your way to correcting those imbalances and then eventually weaning off most products – More about that in moment.

Right now, I'd actually like to share with you the "Top 15 Nutritional Supplements" prescribed by Naturopathic, Medical, Osteopathic, and Chiropractors[17]:

TOP 15 PRESCRIBED SUPPLEMENTS

1. Digestive Enzymes
2. Magnesium
3. Vitamin D3
4. Probiotics
5. Activated B-Complex
6. Glutamine
7. Adrenal Adaptogens
8. Prenatal Vitamin
9. NAC (n-acetyl cysteine)
10. Activated Multi-vitamin
11. Curcumin
12. All-In-One Shake
13. Omega-3
14. Vitamin K
15. CoQ 10

I reviewed the cross-disciplinary lists multiple times and couldn't believe the overlap from health practitioners all over the country. These doctors can prescribe anything they want in terms of nutritional supplements, but these same ones kept coming up!

This is *no coincidence.*

The list you're looking at above has a mountain of scientific data proving each one's efficacy. A simple *Google Scholar, PubMed,* or *National Standard Database* search will bring up thousands of scientific studies for each supplement listed.

The other interesting note I took away from reviewing this research was that almost anyone could take the items listed above and receive tremendous benefit.

The issue is that's a lot of pills to take, it can be expensive, and for the most part I only believe in taking the minimum amount of nutritional supplements needed to keep you healthy and strong.

DECIDING ON WHAT TO TAKE

It can be hard to decide which supplements to take. There are so many with sound scientific research that you may want to take them all in hopes of achieving your end goals of wellness, weight loss, and anti-aging.

However, it's my opinion that besides using a good quality activated multi-vitamin or all-in-one shake, it's best not to begin using a handful of supplements all at once. The reason I say this is because it's better to see how each one affects you before adding another.

My one exception to this rule is if you completed Functional Medicine testing to find out which vitamins, minerals, or other nutrients you are deficient in.

Personally, I have my wellness clients run an Organic Acids Test to look at their vitamin levels and a Hair Tissue Mineral Analysis to find out their mineral levels. By doing this I can customize a nutritional supplement protocol specifically for their needs.

You can have access to these same tests and discover your own nutritional needs by completing these labs right at home. You may also be able to find a qualified Functional Medicine practitioner or doctor in your area to run them, or simply go to StephenCabral.com/rbe for direct links to those labs and many others.

USING NUTRITIONAL SUPPLEMENTS

After initially helping someone to get well and rebalance their body (typically 12-16 weeks) I begin to wean them off most of their recommended nutritional supplements.

Usually, I'll simply recommend an organic fruit and vegetable greens powder, an all-in-one shake or activated multi-vitamin, and potentially a probiotic. If their omega-3 levels tested low, I will also keep them on a quality Omega-3 product tested to be free of oxidation and heavy metals like mercury. And, in the Winter (or if levels are low) I will add vitamin D3 for immunity, hormones, heart health, mood, and so much more.

There are obviously exceptions like taking additional calcium/magnesium, b-vitamins, adaptogens, etc., but unless someone enjoys taking nutritional supplements I typically opt for just the "big 3" I mentioned above.

Since I get asked quite often, I'll share my personal maintenance plan.

"THE DR. CABRAL DAILY PROTOCOL"

I've been using this same morning routine for over 4 years. I've honestly never felt better, been healthier, or had more energy in my life.

My private wellness clients have enjoyed the same results, which is why I want to share it with you now. The reason why it works so well, is that it's a combination of both whole food and Functional Medicine nutrition.

It supplies over 100% of the RDA for vitamins, minerals, and antioxidants, so you're assured to get everything you need right at breakfast each day. Again, I like to refer to it as my "safety net."

Originally, I created it for busy people on the run and for those that didn't want to take supplements throughout the day. I had to come up with something that would combine everything first thing before their hectic day got started.

Here's what I created:

The cornerstone is a breakfast smoothie using my Daily Nutritional Support Shake. This is a Functional Medicine hypoallergenic, vegan organic protein powder that also contains a full multi-vitamin, mineral, antioxidant, electrolyte, and gentle detox support.

In addition to this, I use 1 serving of my Daily Fruit & Vegetable Blend. This is 22 organic fruits and vegetables in powdered form. It is gluten, dairy, soy, egg, and nut free. It provides the best of fruit and vegetable nutrition to make up for the fact that most people don't eat a wide variety of produce on daily basis.

Finally, I maintain healthy gut flora with my Daily Probiotic Support. This is a dairy-free, low histamine probiotic that's meant to keep the intestinal microbiome clean and balanced.

It works exceptionally well even for the most sensitive digestive system because it was formulated for just that reason. It also provides 50 Billion CFU, which you can take right before breakfast or with your smoothie.

That's it – Just enjoy one powerful smoothie to have as breakfast, or along with your current breakfast, and it will provide every vitamin, mineral, and nutrient your body needs to stay healthy and strong.

It's also great to know that even if someone doesn't eat particularly well for the rest of the day they've at least consumed all the fruits, veggies, vitamins, minerals, and other nutrients their body needs to function optimally.

On the resource page for this book, I also provide a free smoothie recipe guide that has over a dozen smoothie and green juice recipes. My long-time favorite has been the "Purple Crush Smoothie," made with frozen high-antioxidant wild blueberries – It's delicious!

Lastly, although those 3 nutritional supplements do make up the cornerstone of my wellness maintenance protocol, I do add in other supplements daily. Typically, I'll use a b-vitamin during times of higher stress, magnesium for deeper sleep at night, and adrenal adaptogens when traveling, etc.

Honestly, I'm always investing in high-quality products of all types to continue to keep my body feeling great!

ONE WORD OF CAUTION

After just espousing the virtues and benefits of nutritional supplements I feel obligated to also share the dark side of this industry.

Every year tens of millions of dollars in counterfeit nutritional supplements are sold online. I'll give you one guess which site they're sold on – If you guessed Amazon.com, congratulations you are correct.

Like any industry that has the power to help a lot of people, there will also be people that have no morals and are simply looking to cash in on what's hot. This means you could be being scammed right now in 1 of these 4 ways:

WHITE POWDER

Since so many products are clear vegetable capsules with white powder inside, there are counterfeiters that simply add baking soda or other fillers to those capsules and pass them off as the real deal. Although this isn't particularly dangerous (assuming it's baking soda), you're also paying money for a fake product.

The other issue is that scammers are creating their own fake labels for companies you would otherwise know and trust. This means everything looks the same as it would when purchasing from your favorite company except for the fact that the product is counterfeit. The only way you would know the difference is to look for the *batch stamp* on the bottom.

EXPIRED SUPPLEMENTS

Often times a supplement company will sell products at a deep discount close to their product's expiration date. This allows the end consumer to get a good deal and the company ensures they don't lose money on inventory they can't move in time.

The issue is that people will buy the supplement bottles in bulk and then scratch off the expiration date which is stamped in ink. After that, they stamp their own new "made-up expiration date" and resell it online. So now you're paying for old supplements that have either gone bad or do not have the same potency.

BOGUS CLAIMS

Once an online marketer sees that a certain product is selling well, they will typically knock that competitor's product off. This means they'll copy as much as they can of the popular supplement. However, they need to undercut the price of the best-selling product, so they source cheaper ingredients.

Typically, this means using non-activated (absorbable) versions of vitamins and cheap forms of minerals.

For example, folic acid is very inexpensive, whereas the more absorbable and safe form called NatureFolate of methylfolate (5-MTHF) is more expensive. Another example that is common is using calcium carbonate, which is a poorly absorbed and potentially dangerous version of this mineral instead of using a more absorbable form like calcium citrate.

Unfortunately, many women unknowingly take this product every day.

INEFFECTIVE DOSES

Another popular tactic of online marketing supplement companies is to piggy back off the latest research to advertise their products.

They'll mention a claim based on an ingredient in their product and show you how you'll get a certain benefit based on real research.

The problem is that the clinical research may have used a dosage of let's say 3,000mg of omega-3 oil and the marketing company's product only contains 600mg. Are they using the same ingredients? Yes, but the product will be most likely ineffective due the fraction of the dosage used in research.

Essentially, all of the devious tactics used above are all to gain market share and create the lowest cost supplement with the highest margins. These companies *do not care* about the end consumer. They simply want to fill their pockets with profits at the expense of everyone.

Plus, these same companies create fake Amazon (or website) reviews to boost their product to the top and make it look like they're highly effective. You won't believe this, but they actually teach entire seminars on how to do exactly that – it's deceptive and deplorable!

This is why I recommend always purchasing from your local health practitioner or home town health food store whom gets their products directly from the supplement manufacturer.

If you do order online it should be directly from the manufacturer (same company name as on the bottle) or from a qualified natural health practitioner's or doctor's website that you trust. And remember, if you ever see a supplement that costs much less than others in the same category there's always a reason why – Be careful.

Understand that good quality nutritional supplements cost a lot to make and trying to save a few dollars in this area is not the best place to try and save money.

I also believe that by choosing just a handful of high quality Functional Medicine backed supplements only, you should be able to keep your supplement budget to $5 a day total (about the same as a Starbuck's latte) and still get the vitamins, minerals, and nutrients your body needs.

WHY NOT JUST EAT A GOOD DIET?

I get this question all the time, so I wanted to answer it here.

I used to be an idealist and believe that I could get all my nutrition through a whole food's diet. The problem was that most studies don't back that up.

As I stated earlier, not only is it near impossible to get every nutrient your body needs even with an organic, whole foods, predominantly plant-based diet. Plus, eating that much organic food is typically cost prohibitive for most people.

Besides all the other countless reasons such as depleted nutrient levels in soil, polluted oceans, polluted air, fertilizers with negative impacts on produce, overfished seas, pesticides on fruits/vegetables, diseased animals, and hormone loaded dairy products, there's one big reason that made me abandon my food only approach…

The issue was that as I started to see case after case of digestive disorders, auto-immune diseases, fatigue, skin issues, and everything else you could imagine, I began to realize that many of these people were already eating well and following some type of elimination diet.

Yet, they still weren't well or able to lose weight!

And if that were the case, how could I realistically expect them to get dramatically different results with just a few small food tweaks?

I couldn't and that's when I realized 3 major issues that plague most people who are feeling sick, overweight, or just have a case of the "blahs."

WEAK DIGESTION

One of the reasons why it simply doesn't matter if a person is eating the best foods in the world, is because if their digestion is weak they can't fully break down and absorb the nutrients in even the best organic, non-GMO foods. As stated previously, this is due to either being on an acid-blocking drug, stress, poor food combining, or other factors.

Ultimately, it leads to poor stomach acid balance, low bile production, and an imbalance of gut bacteria, which I'll speak about in a moment.

This is why, in the beginning, nutritional supplements will actually be better absorbed than hard to digest foods. In almost all cases, I also recommend a daily digestive enzyme formula and a cup of ginger tea with meals to compensate for about the first 12 weeks.

A POLLUTED GUT

Gut dysbiosis, which means an imbalance in bad to good gut bacteria (probiotics or flora) is a massively overlooked cause of most mental and physical health issues.

Once you realize that there are more bacteria in your gut than there are cells in your body, you will begin to understand the importance of this synergistic relationship.

One of the reasons I've been so successful at helping people overcome their health and weight issues is because of the gut balancing protocols I've been fortunate to see work in my practice. The candida, bacterial overgrowth, parasite and gut rebuilding protocols I've been able to develop have literally *transformed* the lives of people who once suffered from the worst dis-eases you can imagine.

I feel grateful to have discovered them by studying all over the world and it's also why I show you on my website exactly what I use. Then, I give you the option of purchasing them anywhere in the world you would like.

For me, I already feel blessed for the way nutritional supplements have helped me overcome my wellness issues and gave me my life back. My mission now is to simply share what I've learned with the world. I know for many, healing the gut is most likely the first place to start.

DIRTY BLOOD

Polluted gut flora creates an inflamed and infected intestinal tract, which can eventually lead to leaky gut. When this happens, the actual bacteria, candida, parasites, pathogens, and undigested food particle waste can move directly into the blood stream.

Leaky gut syndrome leads to an exaggerated immune response in order to clean the blood of these "intruders."[18] It also forces the liver to work harder in phase 1 and 2 detox in order to remove the toxins. So, although your liver is always working to filter the "dirt and debris" from your blood it can become overwhelmed.

This is why nutritional supplements used in detoxification are vitally important. Your liver cannot function properly, or to full capacity, without specific vitamins, minerals, and amino acids. The problem is very few doctors knows this, so they can't share it with you.

Essentially the bottom line is that most of us have been sold a false narrative telling us that our bodies run just fine regardless of what we put in them... I've even heard some doctors go so far as to say that "no matter what breaks, they always have a surgery or drug to fix it!" I find this type of rationale irresponsible and egotistical. Why not try to help people before they become sick and have to suffer a life-time of chronic disease or surgeries?

If more time was taken to educate the world on the benefits of good quality, research-driven, Functional Medicine supplements, I believe 99% of all health conditions could be reversed. The reason I say this is due to the fact that nutritional supplements do not cure disease. They don't have any effect on any disease. That's because *a disease is only a name we choose to give a specific set of symptoms.*

Therefore, if you use a protocol that helps to rebalance your body and Empty Your Rain Barrel™ of built up toxicities and vitamin and mineral shortages that have contributed to your symptoms, you can no longer experience the disease itself. Remember, a healthy balanced body cannot be sick, overweight, or unhealthy!

Before we get into our last section of the DESTRESS Protocol™ I want to provide you with a straight forward action plan to get started on using high-quality nutritional supplementation the right way.

EMPTY YOUR RAIN BARREL™ SUPPLEMENT PROTOCOL

Besides beginning to put healthier foods into your body that contain less toxins, I'd be remiss if I didn't share what I do to help people all over the world live healthier happier lives. You have 2 approaches when beginning to take nutritional supplements:

1. PERSONALIZED WELLNESS PLAN

This approach allows you to work with a Natural Health Practitioner of Doctor and run a few Functional Medicine lab tests to see what your vitamin and mineral levels are. You can also run lab tests to look at digestive function if you suspect issues. This will enable you to personalize what your body needs the most. You can work with our Functional Medicine (FM) practice over Skype anywhere in the world, or seek out a FM practitioner near you. The lab tests mentioned earlier are linked up at StephenCabral.com/rbe

2. START WITH THE BASICS

Before you get to adding in more superfood powders, turmeric, Co-Q10, isolated B-12, maca, or any one of the popular supplements of the day, my highest recommendation is to follow the Dr. Cabral Daily Protocol as shared in this chapter. It costs about the same as a typical breakfast, yet it guarantees you every vitamin, mineral, and nutrient your body needs to repair, rebuild, and rejuvenate itself. Most people will never need more than this to maintain optimal mental and physical health & well-being.

(Note: Since I know there's always the occasional cynic saying that natural health doctors are trying to promote one supplement or another, I always provide 3rd party distributors on the resource page. The choice is always yours of where to buy. I just want to make sure you get the help you need to take back control of your own body and enable you to follow the same protocols I see work every day in my practice!

Success (Mindset)

Growing up I always accepted what my parents, teachers, and the government said was the way things were.

In the beginning, this helps to give you some guidance, but in the long-run it's not the best formula for success.

No one is infallible and it turns out that when we were little the "adults" were mainly passing down what was taught to them. And, if their upbringing or experiences weren't the most positive, you might have been passed on some messages that may conflict with your ideal vision of the world as well.

I was told, like most people, to accept what my doctor told me as "divine truth." Who was I to challenge the brilliance of a medical doctor?

So, I didn't… This left me shuttling from specialist to specialist until I finally gave up. They concluded my illness was psychosomatic (a.k.a. all in my head) because they couldn't find anything wrong with me on my blood work and other labs or my physical exam.

Luckily, my parents also taught me to never give up. It was this will that would eventually allow me to persevere and succeed. It is why I am here today writing this book. It is also with my highest recommendation that I am now asking you to question all of your assumptions up to this point in your life.

If you don't like where you are, then what you're currently doing is not working. The bottom line is that if you want to change, something has to change in your life. This final chapter of the DESTRESS Protocol™ will teach you how to overcome your current struggles and take with you lessons that you can apply to any area of your life.

THE JOURNEY BEGINS NOW

About 20 years ago, I couldn't walk up more than 6 stairs without having to lie down and wait for my heart to stop pounding through my chest.

Conventional medicine called it a form of Postural Orthostatic Tachycardia Syndrome (POTS). This label was in addition to my growing list of dis-eases such as Myalagic Encephalomyelitis, Chronic Fatigue Immune Dysfunction Syndrome, Type 2 diabetes, Addison's Disease, Mastocytosis, GERD, Acid Reflux, Allergies, Autoimmune, Candida Overgrowth, and SIBO.

It's quite the list. And the only answer I was given was that I'd have to be medicated the rest of my life – Conventional medicine had no explanation as to *why* I was suffering like this. The thought of living like a "zombie" for the remainder of my days was excruciating for me. I felt like I was meant to live for more in my life.

This cognitive dissonance of where I was in life and where I wanted to go, left me in state of anxiety and depression. I wanted to give up, and I did many times… But each time after a few days, weeks, or months of feeling sorry for myself, I got angry and I got back up to try to take my body, mind, and life back. I wanted to be more than my current state of health.

THIS SHOULD NOT HAVE HAPPENED

What I'm about to share with you is the end result of successfully turning my life around.

I'm humbled and grateful to say that the life I live now is one I could never have imagined. I feel better now than I did as a teenager. I have more energy, drive, ambition, vitality, and love for life then I can ever remember, *and* it seems to increase each and every year.

By all accounts this shouldn't happen. I was told people don't recover from the "diseases" that I had. I was also taught from a young age that we should decline as we get older.

I'm here to tell you that none of this has to be true for *you*.

TAKE YOUR FIRST STEP TO SUCCESS

I read a book many years ago by Maxwell Maltz, called Psycho-Cybernetics.

In that book, he spoke about how as a plastic surgeon he saw men and women come in with expectations that once they changed their appearance everything in life would change. The problem was, that although their outward looks may have changed, they still held the same limiting beliefs. The result, of course, was that they were still unhappy…

This is why working harder on your mindset than you do your body is always the best place to start. It's simply not possible to overcome many health, weight loss, autoimmune, and other wellness-based issues without first figuring out what your mental roadblocks are.

The first step always begins with you – Always.

I will help guide you and you may even have few close friends or family to support you, but the ultimate responsibility will always lie with you. It has to – Only you have the power to heal you.

It also took me many years to realize no one can or will do the work except for me. I must be the one to take charge because it's my life. Everyone has their own issues to deal with and cannot be responsible for me. Plus, I'm with me 24 hours a day and I have to start liking and accepting who I am, where I currently am, and where I want to eventually be.

A few months ago, I recorded one of our most popular Cabral Concept podcasts to date. During that show, I presented a straight forward 10-step methodology for viewing life from a new perspective. This perspective when followed leads to more happiness, love, forgiveness, and success.

Right now, I'd like to share those 10 steps with you.

YOUR PURPOSE & PATH

Often times success remains elusive only because we've never taken the time to define it. And since happiness, success, and enjoyment in life are subjective, only you can decide what success means to you.

What I've found on my own journey back to health, as well as with working with thousands of others is that those that are most happy and fulfilled seem to be focused on something outside of themselves. They have a great mission or purpose. Oftentimes, this purpose is one of service whether it be through a business, a muse, an art, a passion, trying to be the best parent they can be, or anything that holds their fascination.

Some of the best artists and CEOs I know seem to get lost for hours when working on their craft. Time almost seems to stand still. They love it. It's this type of passion that wakes people up with energy in the morning without an alarm clock, fills their day with worthy challenges, and keeps depression at bay.

I urge you to take some quiet time alone and look at your life from an objective standpoint to see what it is that gives you that kind of passion and purpose. Try to give this passion of yours more of your attention as you're beginning to learn how to get more out of life. Passion for hobbies, your work – These are so important for keeping you really excited about being alive and wanting to live longer so you can enjoy every day of your life.

UNREALISTIC EXPECTATIONS

When I first got sick, I thought I could recover once I found the right doctor that had the right pill. I assumed that there had to be some type of medication to flip the switch on my dis-ease and return me back to my old self.

This mindset – One of a cure that only required medication, and no healthy action on my part, led me to jump from doctor to doctor for a long time. However, even after I followed what is now the DESTRESS Protocol™ and I got fully well, I still suffered for many months believing I still hadn't made it.

The issue was that I believed every single day was supposed to be a "perfect 10." If had the slightest bit of fatigue, a little sniffle, or if I wasn't all smiles, I thought something was wrong. I didn't realize that that's not how life and our body and mind work.

My own limiting belief was that I hadn't yet "made it," until every day I would feel so energized and happy it would feel like I had won the lottery. When you have this kind of mindset, you're setting yourself up to fail. You've missed the point that we as humans are not static beings. We are constantly adapting to our mental and physical environment.

Some days will always be better than others… And that's okay!

THE HUMAN EXPERIENCE

After I studied thousands of hours of ancient philosophy, psychology, and different viewpoints on the world, I began to realize that the unrealistic expectations I had were also part of this journey we're all on.

I began to innately understand that all the great philosophers and speakers alluded to a certain "ebb and flow" to life. Meaning, we go through highs and lows. Jim Rohn, one of my favorite motivational teachers, referred this these times in our life as "the seasons."

We have the winter, when things often seem depressing and barren, but then comes the spring where small signs of life begin to glimmer. If we take hold of these signs, we can then pull ourselves up and work to improve our life during our summer cycles. As the fall comes, we enjoy what we have worked towards while knowing now from experience that we must prepare for another winter.

I used to resent this thought of ever having to endure hard times. Finally, though, I saw the wisdom in it. I realized that even the "hard times," don't have to be so bad as long as we understand, they too, are part of this human experience we are all joined together on.

It's also helpful to know that no matter how bad you have it right now, spring will come – just look for the signs and then act upon them.

ASK FOR MORE OUT OF LIFE

I've come to realize that what I was taught in schools and by my community when I was growing up, is almost criminal.

I was led to believe like most people that there are rich people and poor people, smart people and not-so-smart people, healthy people and sick people, and so on – That's just the way it is. You were either born into a certain class, body, intelligence, or you weren't.

You're taught there's basically not much you can do from there. Maybe you can get slightly ahead, but don't ask for too much more than that. You'll only be setting yourself up for disappointment "they" say…

This cultural mental prison keeps people from ever really fully experiencing life. It forces dreams to remain unrealized. When this happens, a part of us goes dark inside. I believe many of us feel we are destined for more – That we deserve more out of life.

If you believe you are one of those people, I urge you to never give up on your dreams. Dreamers are happier, more playful, and fulfilled. They believe in themselves and their potential. This is the first step to taking charge of your life…

YOU NEED TO ASK THE RIGHT QUESTIONS

One of the reasons we never achieve our goals is that we're told to take everything at face value.

For example, if you have an autoimmune dis-ease, you've been told your immune system is simply "malfunctioning." We now know this is not true. We've seen the research prove that 90%, if not all, autoimmune diseases have gut-based issues as a root cause.[1]

Another example would be being told you'll just have to take insulin the rest of your life if you're type 2 diabetic. Again, this is simply not true. By changing your nutrition, sleep, exercise, cell membrane health, and reregulating the way your body uptakes sugar you can reverse your type 2 diabetes in many cases.[2]

This list goes on and on, but in the majority of cases, most people have been brainwashed into believing that there is only one way to be successful at achieving your goals. Be it health, career, relationships, etc., you must begin to think differently.

You must be constantly asking yourself, "What am I missing? What questions should I be asking in order to achieve my goal? What have other people in my current position done in order to turn their life around? How can I copy their success, so that I too can get those same results?"

Often times, success lies in the quality and quantity of uncomfortable questions we're willing to pose to our self…

TAKE THE BULL BY THE HORNS

I get emails from people all over the world from outside of my practice, asking me why they still aren't well yet. They go on to name a half dozen or so diet plans, or nutritional supplements they've tried.

I then go on to ask them how long they did each one? Did they take any worthwhile data from that previous experience? Did they then build off of it when moving to the next plan? Are they still continuing to move forward?

You see, part of the issue is that we don't give things enough time to actually manifest. We live in an immediate gratification society where we expect to get all the results we want within a week or two. The problem is our bodies (and minds) don't work that way. It takes repetition, the creation of new rhythms, and often a few months for more serious conditions to begin to clear up.

My recommendation is to never give up. Push forward. Learn from your mistakes and try not to repeat them. Seek out mentors, coaches, and trainers to help you learn and grow. It's your body and it's the only one you've been given. You're worth the time and effort it will take in order to get well, lose the weight, and finally feel alive again!

YOU CAN DO ANYTHING

Sometimes you feel that the odds are stacked against you…

Maybe everyone in your family has an auto-immune issue, cancer, dementia, or is obese. Maybe it's all you've ever been around and it's all you know. All of that may be true, but it doesn't have to remain that way.

As I've stated before, lifestyle and environment account for 95% of all good or poor health. Genetics do matter, but they are just a small part of the equation. Our thoughts and actions as input devices are what matter most.

If you start to believe that you can achieve anything you set your mind to, everything will change for you. You will see possibility where there were once only obstacles that stood in your way. For every story you could tell me of how hard you have it, I can assure you there are an equal number of stories of people that overcame those same hardships and are now living the life you've always dreamed of.

I'm not saying your situation is a good one right now. I understand where you're coming from – I've been there. However, I need you to stop places limits on yourself of what you can be or achieve. You can be, do, and have anything you want in this life.

YOU ARE THE SUM OF ALL YOUR CHOICES

There are no overnight successes.

It's romantic to think that like in the movies someone gets snatched up from sickness or obscurity and pops right into the life they've always imagined. The issue, of course, is that that's a Hollywood movie, not real life.

In real life, our current condition is the result of millions of small choices (and some larger ones) that have created this state you're living in. It may not be a happy or healthy one, but then again, you may have been unknowingly living on "autopilot" and not really thinking about what thoughts and actions you've been taking.

You see, our thoughts and actions begin to snowball overtime. They start small and insignificant, but with enough momentum they grow. This eventually overflows your rain barrel and you see for the first time what you've become.

It may be an illness, weight gain, a mood disorder, or an overall poor quality of life. You didn't see it coming, but then again you couldn't have for you didn't know this principle:

You are the sum of every action you take.

It is these accumulated thoughts, beliefs, and actions that shape your life into something worth living – Or not. The great thing about this is that at any point *you can change course.*

You can begin to think and act differently. You can begin to accumulate new healthy thoughts and actions. You can recreate your life starting right now *one moment at a time.*

STOP PROCRASTINATING

After explaining some of these principles to people they begin to become overwhelmed with possibilities. They don't know where to start. They get what's referred to as "paralysis by analysis" where they choose to do nothing due to information overload.

This is why it's important to step back and simply realize the next path you take may not be perfect either. It's actually highly unlikely it'll be the "magic bullet" you've been looking for. But, it's the exact next step you do need to take. For without it, you won't be able to then learn from it and move on to the next. It is each subsequent step in life that leads to the growth we've been searching for.

Therefore, since you now know that being perfect or getting it "just right" isn't even an option, there's no need to procrastinate. It's just time to put your head down and get to working towards the realization of your goals. So once you've figured out what you believe to be the best course of action for you, don't second guess it. Take action, move forward, and readjust as needed along the way.

HAVE FUN

Sometimes, when we're discussing serious matters such as taking back our health, body, or mind, we lose track of something . . .

We fail to realize our time on this earth is short — *really* short. As you get older, this realization becomes frighteningly obvious. The holidays come faster and faster and you see people all around you getting older.

Even as young 20-something year old, still not fully well, I decided one sleepless night that I was no longer going to suffer. I said to myself "I'm going to keep some hope alive that I will get well, but I don't know if it will ever happen. Either way, though, I'm not going to live my life depressed."

That night was a turning point.

From that point on, I gave myself daily (and sometimes hourly) pep-talks that my dis-ease did not define me. I was going to have fun and love life no matter what. To me this "fun" meant enjoying life to the fullest. I started creating travel plans, a new career path, relationship goals, and investing in new hobbies.

It turned it out that forcing myself to have a little fun was great medicine. It was contagious. This new mindset led to me opening up my mind to additional possibilities. I ended up being introduced to forward thinking health practitioners that I may never have been open to meeting if I was stuck in my "woe is me state."

The bottom line is that no one knows how long they're given on this earth. We must literally cherish each day. Tomorrow isn't promised to anyone, so please *do try to look for the joy in life*, and if necessary, do what I did and force yourself to "have fun" and just smile. It may just be the tipping point you needed to turn your life around.

I go far more in depth on the podcast, but I hope those 10 steps began to open your mind for how to view life differently. Remember, our mind is intimately connected to our body. Our thoughts give our body life, or drain it of energy. At some point, conventional medicine is going to have acknowledge this connection in order to help people fully heal.

Now I want to help you develop an actual plan for putting everything together.

THE SMART FORMULA

I believe it's my job as an integrative doctor to incorporate the best of everything.

So when I found out that in the corporate world they teach a goal achievement formula that nearly guarantees success, I knew I had to apply it in my Functional Medicine practice. Truth be told, though, this formula can be applied to any area of your life.

Right now, I'd like to give you an example of how my team and I help body transformation clients achieve their goals using the SMART success formula (you can also use it for health and happiness).

SPECIFIC

The first letter in the formula stands for specific. It refers to the need for defining exactly what your goal is. Using our weight loss example, we work with each client to define what their target body fat percentage, weight, or body shape looks like. We then put a number to it. In this example, I'll refer to Janet whose *specific* goal was to lose 32 lbs. This was her "pre-baby weight" and she wanted to get back to that number on the scale.

MEASURABLE

The "M" stands for measurable. This is where we take the specific goal and then ask how can we use daily, weekly, or monthly data to track progress. This is essential because without doing this step we don't know if we're making headway. In Janet's case, we knew that we could *measure* her progress and create twice a week weigh-in reports of how she was doing based on losing 32 lbs on the scale.

ATTAINABLE

After you decide if your goal is measureable you'll then want to ask if it's attainable. Janet needed to figure out what she must do in order to achieve the results she wanted. She knew she had exhausted her own efforts and that she couldn't do it on her own. She had tried dozens of other diets and workouts, but nothing was working for her. It was at this point that she knew that she must hire a coach or follow a specific program where other people just like her got *attainable* results based on real world success stories.

REALISTIC

The next step in the formula asks the question of whether your specific goal is realistic. In this case, we knew we could help her lose the 32 lbs. even though she had been trying for quite some time and hadn't achieved her goal. We simply had the background and experience to draw upon in order to help her reach her desired end result. Since we had helped thousands of clients like her before and could see what she was missing, we knew that she could do it too. Therefore, her goal was *realistic*.

TIMELY

The last part of the SMART formula focuses on creating a timeline. Our initial body transformation programs are 12-weeks long. Although Janet expressed an interest in continuing to work with our fitness professionals for longer than that, she wanted to get rid of the 32 lbs. in 12 weeks. She knew that she would be more focused with a specific timeline.

Therefore, we helped her formulate a weight loss calendar. To make her goal of losing 32 lbs. in 12 weeks more manageable we divided 32 by 12 and calculated that she would need to lose 2.7 lbs. per week. Now, she could do Monday and Friday weigh-ins to measure her progress and ensure she stayed on track.

The amazing thing about using this SMART Formula is that *just the act* of going through the 5 steps really focuses you on what you need to do to really accomplish your goals. I've seen absolutely amazing success stories come out of using this method and I do hope you give it a try.

I'm also happy to say that Janet lost the 32 lbs. in just under 12 weeks and is thrilled to have her body back! She continues to train and keep her metabolism boosted while improving the overall tone of her body. These same results can be yours and they can be applied to other areas of your life by implementing your own SMART formula.

SUSPENDING DISBELIEF

At some point your brain may actually begin to put up a wall. Although the evidence is there that you can get well, lose the weight, or live a happier healthier life, it starts to create barriers to attaining those goals.

The little voice in your head begins to say that it all sounds good, but it just won't work for you – That you're different. The problem is that "that difference" only exists in your mind.

This is why I'm going to need you to "suspend disbelief." This means that when your logical mind is telling you that this may all sound well and good, there's no way it will work for you, that you must cancel out those thoughts. You must believe you can copy the success of others – Even when you feel you've tried it all before.

It's at this time that I need you to take a deep breath. Relax your nervous system and allow the tension to drop out of your shoulders and chest. Once you're relaxed, I'd like you to then make the commitment to believe in yourself. I'm not even asking for you to believe in me, my plan, or my hopes for you – I just want you to *believe in you.*

The first step, is always believing in you. You must reach down deep and create a feeling that you can get well, lose the weight, or rejuvenate a worn out body. It can happen, but it all starts with a single small belief.

That belief will eventually grow and become so strong that it continues to propel you forward even with every obstacle you may encounter along the way. No path to success is a straight line, but then again if it were that easy you would have already achieved your goals. You know it's going to take just a bit more effort. But I think you also know it's going to be worth it…

At first, this belief in yourself will take some constant repetition, some self-pep talks and a few back and forths with that little voice, but eventually it will set in. There's actually a name for this initial stage of where you're not a true believer yet. It's called the "fake it until you make it" period.

FAKE IT UNTIL YOU MAKE IT

Before anyone achieves anything worthwhile, they have to "pretend" they've already been there or done that. This is what gives you the confidence to actually take the first step. It's a bit like playing dress-up, or make believe.

During this stage you need to be asking yourself what would your life look like when you do get well or lose the weight? What will you do then that's different from what you're currently doing? What clothes will you be wearing? What activities might you be doing? Who will you be hanging around with more? How will you feel?

Once you begin to answer these questions it's then time to act. I need you to actually start down the path of that person you envisioned that has already achieved your goal. This means following a plan like the one I've laid out for you in this book, begin an exercise program, make changes to your diet, begin to get more sleep, detox your body, and learn to implement a few key lifestyle changes.

Essentially, I need you to live the life you believe a person would need to in order to achieve the goal you've set for yourself. After all, goals simply don't materialize themselves without someone taking specific action. I want you to go about these actions confidently already assuming your end result will be there after you've done the needed tasks.

There's no magic to this protocol and I can speak firsthand that it certainly beats dwelling on the negative results you're currently experiencing in your life!

BE CONSISTENT

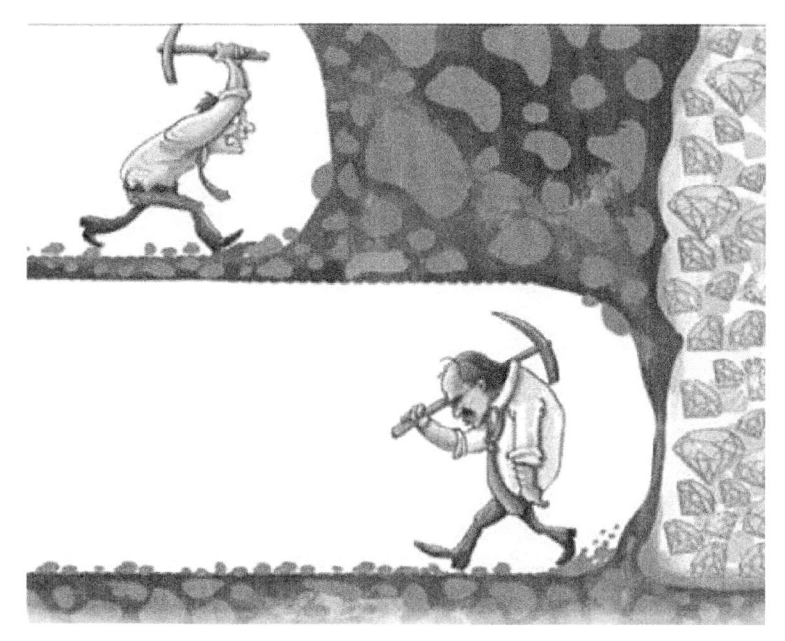

(Don't make it a race to get to your goals, but at the same time be consistent and don't ever give up – You could be just a few "shovels" away from achieving your desires! Photo credit: David McElroy)

Once of the biggest mistakes I see in natural health and weight loss is the misconception that we need to see an immediate turn around within days or a week. If we don't get that result, we think we're on the wrong path.

You're not. You've just been sold a poor philosophy in our "pill for every ill" society. We're so programmed to believe that whenever we go to the doctor they have special pill they can prescribe for every ill we may be experiencing. It's unfortunate, but we carry this same belief through life.

The worst part is that the drugs you're prescribed only mask symptoms. They don't actually work. By that I mean if you were to ever come off the drug, your poor health would re-manifest itself (and often times this eventually happens even if you're medicated).

This scenario clearly defines the difference between conventional and naturopathic medicine. One masks the symptoms and lets the dis-ease fester inside, while naturopathic medicine draws out the root causes and eliminates them permanently. The problem, of course, is that your body takes time to heal at a deeper level. It's not going to happen overnight.

If this frustrates you simply look to nature. Understand that if you plant a fruit or vegetable seed today, it's not going to sprout tomorrow. It may very well take weeks or months, but the end results is worth the wait.

The other good news is this; You don't have to wait months to begin feeling better. Although the deep level work will take time, your symptoms will dissipate much faster. So, you could easily eliminate the symptoms of bloating, digestive issues, pain, etc. within weeks. Also, in my practice, the average weight loss on the Dr. Cabral Detox is 7.2 lbs. in 7 days, 10+ lbs. in 14 days, and 15+ lbs. in 21 days.

As you can see, you can still achieve remarkably quick results with Natural Health. However, as I always like to say, the real work is being done at a deeper cellular level and we must respect this. Your new, fresh red blood cells don't even fully turnover for 120 days. That's why as good as you feel after a few weeks of emptying your rain barrel – In 3-4 months you'll feel like a new person!

97% NEW YOU

You may not know this, but at the end of 12 months you have completely regenerated 97% of your body, even down to your DNA.

This means you're almost a brand new person. It's also why, I believe any person can get completely well, healthy, in shape, and loving life within the next year.

It can be that incredible.

Again, I wouldn't have thought any of this was possible if I didn't first experience it for myself and, then, see it first-hand as I travelled and worked all over the world in various clinics studying under fascinating medical practitioners – And finally, implementing these healing modalities in my practice and watching people's lives change.

PAY IT FORWARD

I have no doubt you will achieve your goals.

You will be successful. Losing weight is actually very achievable when you know the science behind it, and it's made much easier by removing all these toxic variables that stand in your way.

The same goes for getting well. There is always an answer and there is only so deep you can go before finding your imbalances and then correcting them by starting with the DESTRESS Protocol™ explained in this book.

It took me years to find my answers to getting well and another 15 years of reading over 3,000 books and studying all over the world to discover the secrets hidden from our modern world, but now I've made it my mission for the rest of my life to share it with others.

And I'm hoping you'll join me – I am one person and one person can only do so much…

I have this book, my daily *Cabral Concept* podcast, YouTube videos, and website where I teach as much as I can to give back to the world the miracle of health I've experienced. I made a promise many years ago that if I were to ever get well, I would share what I discovered with the world, so I am.

And that's why I'm asking you to *share* what you've learned here.

Your friends, family, and co-workers aren't going to learn it anywhere else. It's not taught in schools and it's no longer handed down from generation to generation, so we have to re-learn what we as a culture have forgotten.

I also believe that the final stage of healing is to pay it forward. I believe there is a deep human need to share with others what you have found to work for yourself. As humans, we're all in this together. You'll find you'll want to share your recovery with others and I highly encourage this. I think you'll also find that by helping to heal another individual, it's a powerfully healing experience for not just them, but you as well.

Personally, I've found that by living and teaching what helped you to finally become successful (in any area of your life), you only reinforce your own results.

THE MOVEMENT HAS ARRIVED

Individually, each one of us holds very little power, but together we cannot be stopped. *Our voices are being heard.*

There is a natural health movement gaining more life every day and each one of us breathes more power into it with every effort to fight back against a broken medical model.

The change is no longer coming – It's already here.

Most people have now become aware of and are seeking "alternatives" to conventional therapies. They understand that masking symptoms *is not* true healthcare. It's at best, a temporary band aid approach.

I urge you now to join this movement yourself. Make it apart of who you are. Begin now, so that you do not look back months or years from now with the regrets of not at least trying. You have the power to change your life.

You really can have it all – but *it starts with first changing your body*.

Once your body is healthy, your thoughts will be clearer, and once your thoughts are clearer, your feelings with be more positive. And once your feelings become more positive, your actions will change for the better, and you will start moving forward with more confidence.

It is at this time you will be well on your way to living the life of your dreams. It's time to get well, lose the weight, and feel alive again!

You now have my entire DESTRESS Protocol™ in your hands that you can begin to implement in your life to Empty Your Rain Barrel™ of the toxins that have built up in your mind and body. Since much of the time it is these toxins that are holding you back from your goals and dreams, I'd like to share with you one more section that I almost left out of the book.

The reason I didn't end up omitting this final chapter is that after careful consideration I wanted to provide you everything I use in my practice so you too could copy the success my private clients get to enjoy. This next section is the exact manual I provide with my Dr. Cabral Detox program. If I could point you in one single place to start to achieve any of your wellness, weight loss, or anti-aging goals this would be it. Enjoy!

EMPTY YOUR RAIN BARREL™ SUCCESS (MINDSET) FORMULA

Use your current state of motivation to begin outlining your own SMART Formula. Try to answer the questions below as a starting point for achieving your first (of many) goals!

1. What SPECIFIC goal do you want to achieve?
2. How will you measure this goal at least weekly?
3. What will you need to get, be, or do in order to make this goal a reality?
4. Has anyone ever achieved this same goal? Is there a book, program, or coach/mentor/doctor you can hire to achieve your goal?
5. What is your deadline for achieving your goal? Is there a specific date you'd like to reach it by? If so, why does this deadline hold meaning for you?

The Dr. Cabral Detox Manual

First, I want to congratulate you on taking the 1st step to a brand new you.

You've already done more than most people ever will and that's to commit to improving your life and reaching your higher potential.

This is going to be a fun & exciting journey and I can't wait for you to join our community of success stories and those sharing your same story. Together, we all help each other to become better.

This final chapter is the exact manual that comes with every 7, 14, or 21-day Dr. Cabral Detox kit. I wanted to include it as a free bonus to this book because I've seen the results of what it can do for people. It's hard to believe, but a this 21-day "challenge" has been the catalyst that has changed more lives than I ever expected.

I want you to enjoy those same wellness, weight loss, or anti-aging results and that is why I've included the manual in it's entirety. Inadvertently, this manual is also a summary of the major points we spoke about in the book.

In this regard, it should serve as a nice recap of everything we've covered. If you want to skip the *Rain Barrel Effect* summary you can move onto where it says, "*How It Works*."

WHAT TO EXPECT

We've covered a lot in this book. And, the first question is typically, "Where do I start?"

It's a great question and that's why I say if you do nothing else in terms of emptying your rain barrel, I can't recommend the 21-day Dr. Cabral Detox enough. Please do keep in mind that you do not need to use my product even though that is what I see work in my practice. Since I do not want this to be a promotion for my particular recommendation, I also provide other 3rd party sources to choose from other products and a complete meal plan and shopping lists.

Although results will vary, when you Empty Your Rain Barrel™ using the Dr. Cabral Detox you will most likely see a rebalancing in:

- Healthy inflammation levels
- Healthy blood sugar levels
- Hormones
- Toxin reduction
- Join pain
- Allergies
- Metabolism & weight
- Digestion
- Brain fog
- Skin appearance
- Energy
- Mood
- Libido
- Sleep

IT'S TIME TO BEGIN

Remember, this chapter does not exclude the DESTRESS™ Protocol we just reviewed. It simplifies the *diet* and *supplement* sections into one easy to follow protocol. From a clinical perspective, implementing these two first will give you the most tangible amount of results the fastest.

You can then use those first wins and build upon them by adding in the exercise, stress reduction, toxin removers, rest, emotional component and success mindset. Some of those easy add-ons can include dry brushing, Epsom salt baths, meditation, walking, and more rest.

The point I'm trying to make is not to allow everything you could do overwhelm you with simply getting started by doing something. And since the Dr. Cabral Detox can be the springboard to seeing the results you want, that is my highest recommendation of where to begin.

THE RAIN BARREL EFFECT

When I was 20 years old sitting in the waiting room of my allergist's office and suffering miserably from red, swollen shut, itchy eyes, post nasal drip, and chest congestion, I picked up an article lying amongst the magazines.

I had already been dealing with allergies most of my life and had read quite a bit on how to heal them. However, this article immediately caught my attention. I didn't know it at the time, but it would trigger a new mindset that would be the beginning of my healing journey.

This article mentioned a phrase I had never once heard uttered by doctors, specialists, or anyone inside the medical community. To this day, it's still rarely talked about…

It's called the *"Rain Barrel Effect."*

What it is and how it eloquently explains how we get sick, age, and lose our vitality is life-changing. Once you know the how and why you got where you are right now, you can then finally begin to heal.

The Rain Barrel Effect is the answer you've been looking for. It explains the "mystery illnesses" like the one I had where your blood work looks fine, but you're still sick and tired. It also answers the question as to why you may have that auto-immune, skin, join pain, headache, or other officially diagnosed disease.

So, without further ado let me introduce you to the biggest concept in natural health and medicine that's very rarely, if ever, talked about…

THE RAIN BARREL EFFECT EXPLAINED

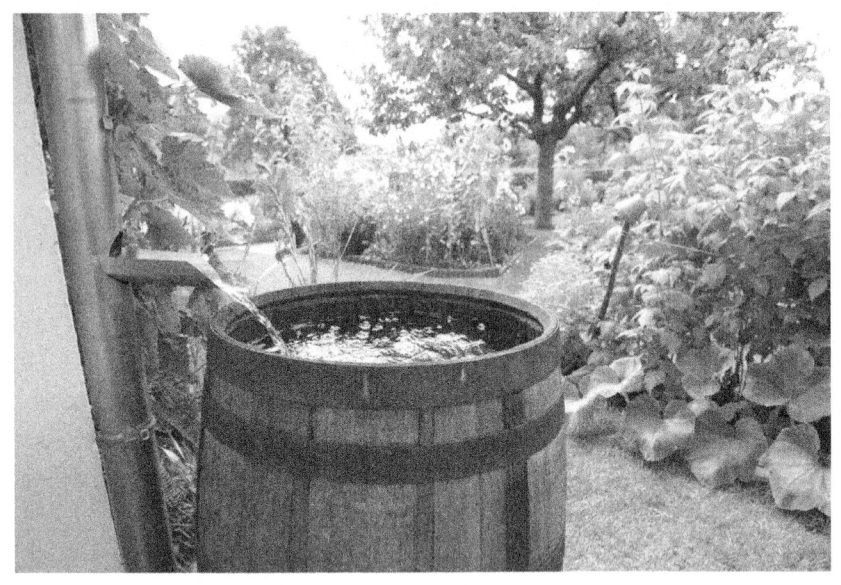

(A rain barrel filling up with waste water from a house gutter)

The best way to think about how and why you got sick, overweight, or just feeling like "blah," is to picture a rain barrel, or just a bucket.

A rain barrel is used to catch water and hold onto it every time it rains. No one ever notices the rain is filling up the barrel. Until of course, the barrel overflows. It's at that point that the barrel needs to be emptied or it will no longer function properly. Instead of the barrel serving a healthy purpose, it will instead spill over onto your garden, patio, or create a dead spot of grass in your backyard.

The same theory holds true for our own bodies. Over time, we accumulate toxins. Some come from the environment and are man-made, such as pollution, pesticides, exhaust fumes, plastics, flame retardants, and heavy metals like mercury and cadmium. Others come from candida, bacteria, parasites, stress hormones, or other internal metabolic processes.

What happens is that when these natural and synthetic toxins float around in our blood is that they must be disposed of. This then takes energy, the proper nutrients, rest, and a well-functioning liver to filter out the harmful substrates. As long as your body is getting everything it needs then the process continues to run smoothly and maintain equilibrium.

ARE YOU MISSING THE SIGNS?

The issue is that as the years pass we accumulate more and more toxins and our bodies begin to run low on certain reserves. Our bodies then begin to lose the internal battle and our rain barrel begins to fill up faster. But, even as your rain barrel is filling up you still may not see any initial symptoms of not feeling well.

The problem is that noticeable external symptoms do not arise until your rain barrel begins to overflow. Unfortunately, just like a real barrel that catches the rain you won't know it's full (unless you lab test) until it's spilling over the sides. The reason for this is that at this point your body, and the barrel, can no longer keep up with the demands placed on it. It does not have enough reserves left.

It's also at this time, that you will begin to feel the outward symptoms of your internal systemic imbalances. You may see or feel pain, skin issues, headaches, fatigue, inflammation, weight gain, a loss in vitality or really any sign of poor health.

You may even be diagnosed with a disease or specific health condition at this point such as high blood pressure, cholesterol, auto-immune, chronic fatigue, fibromyalgia, allergies, asthma, Alzheimer's, Parkinson's, or any other set of symptoms we give a name.

YOU ARE NOT YOUR DISEASE

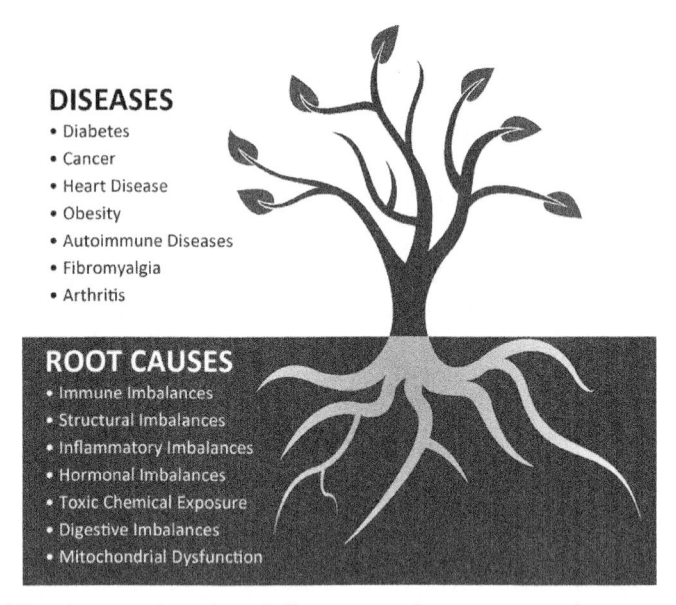

DISEASES
- Diabetes
- Cancer
- Heart Disease
- Obesity
- Autoimmune Diseases
- Fibromyalgia
- Arthritis

ROOT CAUSES
- Immune Imbalances
- Structural Imbalances
- Inflammatory Imbalances
- Hormonal Imbalances
- Toxic Chemical Exposure
- Digestive Imbalances
- Mitochondrial Dysfunction

(This drawing shows how different toxins begin to accumulate in your "rain barrel," which then result in a symptom we call a disease. The medical system then tries to mask those symptoms with medications.)

A rain barrel will of course continue to take on more water, but not without spilling additional contents. It will carry on like this until the owner empties its current load. It has no other choice and neither does your body.

Luckily, just like a *physical* rain barrel, you too metaphorically speaking, can Empty Your Rain Barrel™ and lower your total toxic load!

As I said, when I first learned about this discovery I knew it was going to be an important part of me figuring out how to recover from my own "mystery illness" that the best doctors and specialists in the world couldn't figure out. Little did I know, over a decade later that it wouldn't just play a role in me getting well, it turned out to be the answer that I and many others were searching for...

CHRONIC DISEASE EXPLAINED

No chronic disease, illness, cancer, or any other health issue happens overnight. It is a slow gradual wearing down of our body's defenses that eventually gives way to poor health.

However, what we see is the outcome. We notice the symptoms. And those symptoms such as fatigue, weight gain, join pain, skin issues, infertility, auto-immune, digestive, cancer, etc. are the end results.

The image depicted below is commonly used in Functional Medicine to show patients how they get sick. It also explains to them how they are not their disease. Their disease is merely their body's expression of imbalance and trying to maintain homeostasis within the body.

Each person will always have their own genetic predisposition to what they may have for health issues if their total toxic load becomes too great. For example, in my family everyone gets Rheumatoid arthritis and digestive issues. However, no one seems to get Hashimoto's, Lupus, Multiple Sclerosis or other auto-immune issues.

What's even more interesting is that some new people I see in my practice that come in with an auto-immune issue show me previous lab work where sometimes they had the dis-ease and at other times it wasn't showing up and they were fine. This is called *epigenetics*, which explains how our genes can be turned on and off depending on their environment.

The interesting concept, though, is that these "dis-ease" names are all different expressions from the same malfunctions in the body. We see them as different diseases, but they are not.

They are but different manifestations of an imbalanced body trying desperately to rebalance itself. This is why the symptoms you're dealing with are not the disease itself. Mostly, the symptoms are the outward sign of your body trying to "empty its rain barrel" and rebalance.

For example, most people believe when they get a fever they have to reduce it at the first sign. However, the fever is not the sickness. The fever is your body trying to speed up the flow of white blood cells and raise your core body temperature in order to naturally kill viruses. It is only when a fever becomes too high that we should try to lower it.

Your body knows what it is doing and wants to help you heal. This is why suppressing symptoms will never lead to healing. It can't. The reason is that when you treat the symptoms you are missing the whole point, since the symptoms are a response of the body to an underlying root cause issue imbalance.

IT'S TIME TO EMPTY YOUR RAIN BARREL

This is why I came up with the term, *Empty Your Rain Barrel*™.

I felt that once you knew what the *Rain Barrel Effect* meant, and why we ultimately get sick or gain weight that the next logical step would be to ask, "How do I empty my rain barrel?"

If you're asking that question right now, then you're on the right track to ultimately getting well, losing weight, and feeling alive again! Because without first lowering your toxicity and a lifetime of accumulation, then it's going to be difficult for your body to get back to a state of equilibrium.

So, in real world application, the number one remedy to lowering your total toxic body burden is to complete a simple Functional Medicine detoxification protocol. However, this isn't one of those fruit juice, or maple syrup cleanses. It's not that those are necessarily all bad, it's just that they lack the specific nutrients to truly work with your body's biology.

So, before I literally give you the same protocol I use in my practice, I want to share with you why anyone would decide to complete a Functional Medicine detox protocol…

77,000 REASONS TO DETOX

200 years ago, to get well a simple break from eating and "water fast" would do…

That's because there wasn't the profit seeking, underhandedness of big business looking to cut costs at every corner and as a result create synthetic chemicals to replace natural ingredients. And the fact that they've essentially bought the US Government and many governments around the world, they've passed laws allowing more than 77,000 man-made chemicals into the environment.

Our bodies simply weren't designed for this type of an assault.

As a result, our immune systems and liver are working 24 hours a day trying to clean our blood from the chemicals that enter it through our water, food, air, and the environment around us. But much of the time, our bodies get run down and as a consequence we can't keep up and so the toxins get stored in our fat cells, which cause them to expand. And, inflammation follows right behind as estrogen and cortisol levels rise in both men and women. This also when blood sugar becomes increased due to stress and your cell receptors being blocked…

This is the problem that no one is taking about!

It's not just about eating less and exercising more. That doesn't work anymore. It's also not enough to combat things like chlorine, fluoride, flame retardant materials, bromides in food, BPA, pesticides, preservatives, and tens of thousands of other man-made toxins that pollute our environment and bodies on a daily basis.

This is why it's no longer possible to keep up with the sprayed food & environmental chemicals without some help and support. And that support comes in the form of specific foods and detoxifying supplements to remove these chemicals and purify your body.

HERE'S WHY IT WORKS

If you've never heard of a detox, please don't confuse it with a drug rehabilitation program or anything medical related. Detoxification is a natural function of every human body.

Your body was beautifully designed to have all the blood in your body filtered by your liver (which is an organ located under the right side of your rib cage) every 6 minutes.

Literally, your liver is like your vacuum's filter cleaning everything in your blood 24 hours a day, 365 days a year without a rest!

But, as you can see from the photo above in order for it to do it's job it must get a daily adequate supply of B-vitamins, vitamin C, antioxidants, amino acids and minerals.

And if it doesn't get all those nutrients, the thousands of ducts within your liver can actually begin to get clogged up with bile and toxic sludge-like material that needs to be removed for a healthy functioning body (if not, your skin, energy, mood, weight, sleep, and health will suffer).

Plus, if you only get certain nutrients and not all of those listed, then your liver can't fully complete the detoxification of these harmful toxins by converting them from a fat soluble toxin to a harmless water soluble toxin, which can then be excreted in your urine, stool, or sweat.

This is where most people go wrong. They believe they can still get all the nutrients they need from food alone. I used to believe the same thing, until I realized that most people's digestion is so weak it can't break down all the nutrients your body needs to cleanse itself. To make matters worse, it would take more vegetables than you could possibly eat to get the amount of nutrients needed to fully detox…

THERE IS GOOD NEWS

Since detoxing is actually needed for our very survival, your body always knows what to do to repair itself.

We just need to give it a temporary boost through scientifically researched foods & nutritional supplements that have been proven to assist in liver detoxification and cleaning your blood. After that we let your body take it from there… Remember, we're just here to *support your body*, not tell it how and what to do!

So now that we know why it's so important for everyone to detox and how the natural detoxification process takes place in our body, let's move on to how you're going to easily implement my Dr. Cabral Detox protocol to maximize your results.

6,000 YEAR OLD SECRET REVEALED

Very few people know what I'm about to share with you.

Right now, I'd to share with you one of the most important discoveries for living longer and improving overall health, wellness, and weight loss.

Besides supporting your liver, so that it can better do its job in removing toxins and cancer causing chemicals from your body, there is a process called, *Autophagy*.

It is very well documented now and the research on it actually won the Nobel Prize in Medicine in 2016! How it works is by a process of your own immune system being able to eat up toxins, bacteria, and even cancer cells in your blood like the old video game, "PAC-MAN."

But it can only do that if there are no new substances coming in – And, the only way to do that is to stop eating for a period of time.

The ancient societies and religions all had built-in 24-48 hour fasts during the week (or month). And, Hippocrates, the Father of Modern Medicine, spoke in depth as to how to use fasting as a way to heal the body from the inside out.

Literally, 6,000 years ago in Ayurvedic Medicine they spoke about a rejuvenating process called, "Pancha Karma," that included days or weeks of fasting, a special diet, and detox treatments to heal certain conditions. (I'll be sharing my modern-day version of it up next.)

And, just 70 years ago, Herbet Shelton, one of the original Naturopaths, healed over 35,000 people in his practice, which was centered around water fasting and detoxification.

The results of fasting have stood the test of time and it's literally built into our DNA to fast. The problem is that we have food options around us 24 hours a day and we never go more than a couple of hours between meals without eating (This is not considered a fasting time, since the food is still in your stomach or gut being digested between meals.)

The bottom line is that we're missing out on what is now finally being touted as *one of the greatest healing processes in the world*. After I discovered the benefits of fasting on one of my internships at an Ayurvedic clinic in India, I knew I had to bring this knowledge back to the US and in my clinical practice.

It's also why I specifically designed days 1 & 2 of the Dr. Cabral Detox to include 4 liquid only shakes each day. This allows your liver and body to get the detox nutrients it needs while still keeping the process of autophagy going, so that you get the maximum amount of results without having to strictly water fast.

Remember, you don't need to get overwhelmed with how all this works in order to get results, but I did want to share this amazing breakthrough information with you. Now let's talk about the specifics of how your Dr. Cabral Detox works.

HERE'S HOW IT WORKS

Like every weight loss or wellness plan I design, I try to take complex principles and distill them down to what really matters the most.

There are hundreds of things you could do to lose weight or get well, but there are only a few that actually matter – And, I have no doubt that you are busy and don't have a lot of time to spare. That's exactly why I designed the Dr. Cabral Detox to include very little meal or food prep and you can even take your daily shakes on the go!

To be honest, most people say this plan was one of the most relaxed & enjoyable times of their life, since they didn't really have to think about any of their breakfast meals or all of the typical lunch & dinner choices…

Remember, you've been sold myths in past that have led you to believe that getting well or losing weight has to be a struggle. Nothing could be further from the truth and to be honest, if you need to struggle to get well or take the weight off then you're setting yourself up for failure since it's going to be too difficult to maintain that routine…

Now I'd like to reveal the only 5 things you really need to do in order to lose the weight, get healthy, and improve your overall well-being faster than you ever thought possible.

1. NIGHTLY 12-HOUR OVERNIGHT FAST

Just like it sounds you will be going from 7:00pm - 7:00am without eating or drinking anything except water. You may create any 12-hour time frame you'd like overnight, but try to stop eating 2-3 hours before bed.

2. WHEN TO EAT

To ensure that your body is always getting adequate nutrition and everything it needs to detoxify you will be eating every 3.5 hours beginning approximately 1 hour after waking and ending 2-3 hours before bed.

3. WHAT TO EAT

The Dr. Cabral Detox is simple to use and follow since on days 1 & 2 you are just doing 4 detox shakes per day. Then, on days 3 – 7, you will be having your shake for breakfast, a vegan lunch, another shake mid-afternoon, and finally a vegan, vegetarian, or paleo-style dinner.

4. WHAT TO DRINK

All of your Dr. Cabral Detox shakes should be mixed with 20-30oz of water. This will help keep your hunger away and make sure you are flushing the toxins and fat from your body. Since you'll be getting in at least 10 glasses of water combined with your 4 shakes, you do not need to consume any other liquids if you are not thirsty. However, you may drink as much water (with lemon if you'd like) or herbal tea (ginger tea is best) throughout the day.

Ideally, you will eliminate all coffee, but you may keep in 1 small, black cup in the morning if desired to keep caffeine withdrawal headaches away.

5. REST OR EXERCISE?

If you're not already exercising there's no need to start while on your detox. However, if you're a regular exerciser you may complete your usual routine beginning on Day 3.

It is not recommended that you exercise on Days 1 & 2 (the liquid shake fast days). Please also try to get to bed earlier and allow your body to rest and rejuvenate.

The Dr. Cabral Detox really is this simple to follow and the results will speak for themselves as your friends, family, and co-workers will be wondering what you did to get that new glow.

SIMPLIFIED DETOX EATING PLAN

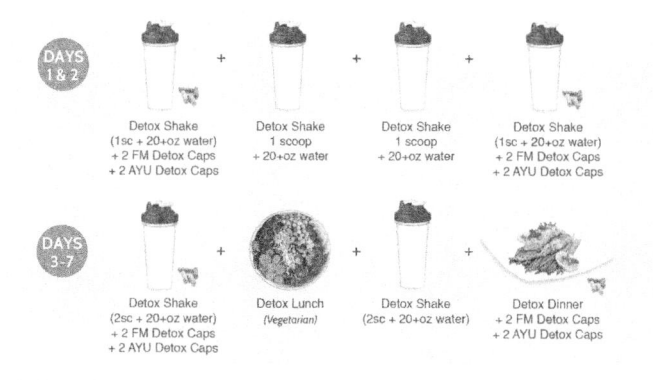

DAYS 1 & 2

Detox Shake (1sc + 20+oz water) + 2 FM Detox Caps + 2 AYU Detox Caps

+

Detox Shake 1 scoop + 20+oz water

+

Detox Shake 1 scoop + 20+oz water

+

Detox Shake (1sc + 20+oz water) + 2 FM Detox Caps + 2 AYU Detox Caps

DAYS 3-7

Detox Shake (2sc + 20+oz water) + 2 FM Detox Caps + 2 AYU Detox Caps

+

Detox Lunch (Vegetarian)

+

Detox Shake (2sc + 20+oz water)

+

Detox Dinner + 2 FM Detox Caps + 2 AYU Detox Caps

(The infographic above outlines the Dr. Cabral Detox meal plan)

As you can see from the image above, the Dr. Cabral Detox is easy to follow and most of our community members say that they felt it was such a relief not to be so focused on where, what, and how to eat for their 7, 14, or complete 21-day detox!

And that's the whole point… I purposely designed the Dr. Cabral Detox to help you begin to reshape your thoughts about eating & nutrition while at the same time giving your body everything it needs to rebalance itself and return to its healthy happy self.

Essentially, the Dr. Cabral Detox is a lot like hitting the reset button on your computer – When things haven't been going well physically, mentally, emotionally, or spiritually the Dr. Cabral Detox allows you to rid your body of the chemicals, heavy metals, toxins, and inflammation holding you back from enjoying the body and mood you deserve.

Lastly, please keep in mind the only thing that will hold you back from being successful on my plan are your limiting beliefs – You can do this, and you will get the same great results as the thousands of community members that you're about to join.

Don't overthink it. The Dr. Cabral Detox has been formulated with the very best ingredients in the world and designed to specifically help those that have been struggling to achieve their wellness or weight loss goals.

MEAL PLANNING MADE EASY

I have to admit, I'm not much of chef.

It's not that I can't follow a recipe, it's just that I don't have the time or interest in cooking elaborate meals. Now, many of our detox members create beautiful and elaborate meals using the foods listed above, but I prefer quick & easy meals to make.

That's why I created this simple "grab & go" meal planning guide.

CREATE DOZENS OF EASY MEALS IN JUST 3 STEPS

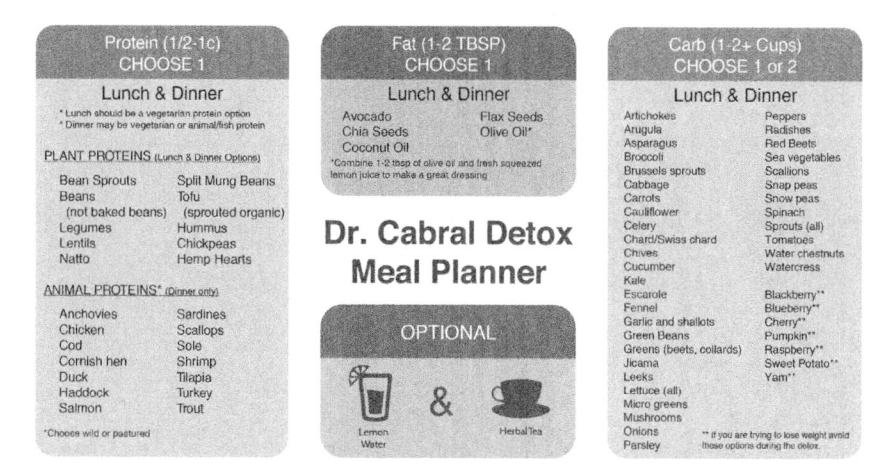

Protein (1/2-1c) CHOOSE 1
Lunch & Dinner
* Lunch should be a vegetarian protein option
* Dinner may be vegetarian or animal/fish protein

PLANT PROTEINS (Lunch & Dinner Options)
- Bean Sprouts
- Beans (not baked beans)
- Legumes
- Lentils
- Natto
- Split Mung Beans
- Tofu (sprouted organic)
- Hummus
- Chickpeas
- Hemp Hearts

ANIMAL PROTEINS* (Dinner only)
- Anchovies
- Chicken
- Cod
- Cornish hen
- Duck
- Haddock
- Salmon
- Sardines
- Scallops
- Sole
- Shrimp
- Tilapia
- Turkey
- Trout

*Choose wild or pastured

Fat (1-2 TBSP) CHOOSE 1
Lunch & Dinner
- Avocado
- Chia Seeds
- Coconut Oil
- Flax Seeds
- Olive Oil*

*Combine 1-2 tbsp of olive oil and fresh squeezed lemon juice to make a great dressing

Dr. Cabral Detox Meal Planner

OPTIONAL
- Lemon Water
- Herbal Tea

Carb (1-2+ Cups) CHOOSE 1 or 2
Lunch & Dinner
- Artichokes
- Arugula
- Asparagus
- Broccoli
- Brussels sprouts
- Cabbage
- Carrots
- Cauliflower
- Celery
- Chard/Swiss chard
- Chives
- Cucumber
- Kale
- Escarole
- Fennel
- Garlic and shallots
- Green Beans
- Greens (beets, collards)
- Jicama
- Leeks
- Lettuce (all)
- Micro greens
- Mushrooms
- Onions
- Parsley
- Peppers
- Radishes
- Red Beets
- Sea vegetables
- Scallions
- Snap peas
- Snow peas
- Spinach
- Sprouts (all)
- Tomatoes
- Water chestnuts
- Watercress
- Blackberry**
- Blueberry**
- Cherry**
- Pumpkin**
- Raspberry**
- Sweet Potato**
- Yam**

** if you are trying to lose weight avoid these options during the detox

(You can download the above shopping list at StephenCabral.com/rbe)

STEP 1: CHOOSE 1 PROTEIN

At lunch and dinner simply choose a handful of your protein of choice. Just make sure lunch is a vegan protein, so that your body has less to detox during the day.

STEP 2: CHOOSE 1 HEALTHY FAT

Adding 1-2 TBSP of olive oil as a dressing is your best choice while on this detox. Please do not cook in any oil.

Oil may be used as a dressing after the food has been cooked or on salads. My favorite dressing is olive oil, a squeeze of lemon, and a pinch of sea salt. You may add herbs such as oregano, thyme, and rosemary.

STEP 3: CHOOSE 2 VEGETABLES (OR MORE)

If you're looking to lose weight, choose any of the vegetables listed above that do NOT have a "*" next to them. The * choices may be included if you do not want the weight loss results, but are still looking for the wellness benefits.

DETOX TIP: LIQUID WITH MEALS

It is best not to drink any water within 30-minutes before a meal and then again for about 1 hour after that meal. (This same digestion rule applies after the detox as well.)

During the meal, sip as little water (with lemon if desired) or ginger tea as possible. And remember, if you've listened to my daily Cabral Concept podcast you already know that you should *never* drink cold water with meals since it will slow digestion and cause bloating.

DETOX TIP: SNACKING?

There is no snacking between shakes, meals, or before bed on the detox.

This will not allow you to give your digestive system a rest between meals. Plus, without pausing to eat between meals you won't allow your body to naturally tap into burning body fat stores and autophagy.

Now that you know how to create your simple detox meals, I want to provide you with a list of "safe" foods to shop for or chose when you're eating out and trying to plan your lunch and dinner options.

Keep in mind you can still grab lunch on the run or go out with friends to your favorite restaurants. You do not have to live the life of a recluse for the next 21 days and close yourself off from the outside world. It's my opinion that we must learn to make healthy choices in every environment.

Using the Detox Food Shopping List below will make it easier to create a healthy lunch or dinner option no matter where you find yourself eating.

DR. CABRAL'S DETOX FOOD SHOPPING LIST

Plant Proteins	Animal Proteins	Carbohydrates	Carbohydrates
☐ Bean Sprouts	☐ Anchovies	☐ Artichoke	☐ Parsley
☐ Beans (not baked)	☐ Buffalo	☐ Arugula	☐ Pepper
☐ Legumes	☐ Chicken	☐ Asparagus	☐ Sea Vegetable
☐ Lentils	☐ Cod	☐ Broccoli	☐ Snap Pea
☐ Natto	☐ Cornish Hen	☐ Brussels Sprouts	☐ Snow Pea
☐ Split Mung Beans	☐ Salmon	☐ Cabbage	☐ Spinach
☐ Tofu (sprouted organic)	☐ Sardines	☐ Celery	☐ Sprouts
☐ Hummus	☐ Scallops	☐ Chard/Swiss Chard	☐ Watercress
☐ Chickpeas	☐ Shrimp	☐ Chives	☐ Daikon Radish
☐ Hemp Hearts	☐ Talapia	☐ Cucumber	☐ Red Beet
	☐ Turkey	☐ Escarole	☐ Tomato
	☐ Trout	☐ Fennel	☐ Carrot
	☐ Wild Game	☐ Garlic & Shallots	☐ Horseradish
		☐ Green Bean	☐ Jicama
		☐ Greens (beet, collard, dandelion, kale, mustard, turnip)	☐ Mushrooms
Fats			☐ Water Chesnut
☐ Avocado			☐ Pumpkin*, Sweet Potato* Yams*
☐ Chia Seeds		☐ Lettuce	
☐ Coconut Oil		☐ Micro Greens	☐ Raspberry*, Blackberry*, Blueberry*
☐ Flax Seeds		☐ Cauliflower	
☐ Olive Oil			

And to make the entire plan just a little easier to visualize, I want to give you one last guide to ensure you understand exactly how the Dr. Cabral Detox works.

SIMPLIFIED MEAL PLAN TIMING
DAYS 1 & 2

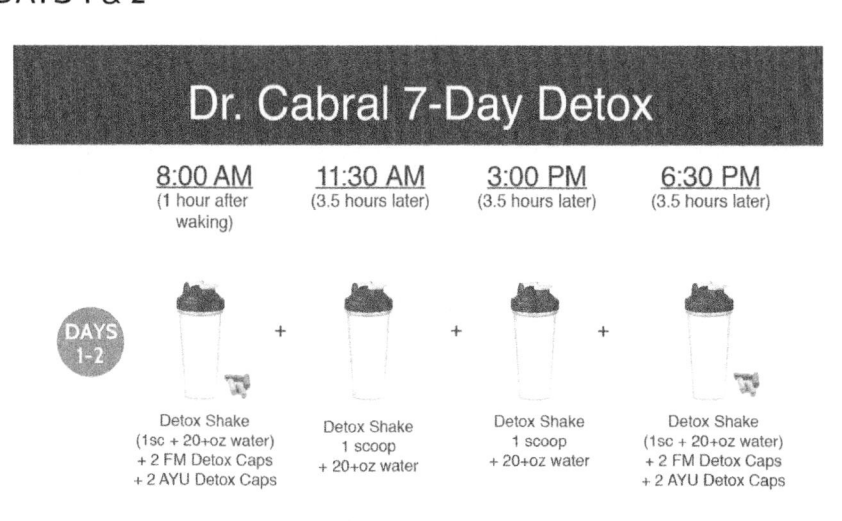

Dr. Cabral 7-Day Detox

DAYS 1-2

8:00 AM (1 hour after waking)
Detox Shake (1sc + 20+oz water) + 2 FM Detox Caps + 2 AYU Detox Caps

+

11:30 AM (3.5 hours later)
Detox Shake 1 scoop + 20+oz water

+

3:00 PM (3.5 hours later)
Detox Shake 1 scoop + 20+oz water

+

6:30 PM (3.5 hours later)
Detox Shake (1sc + 20+oz water) + 2 FM Detox Caps + 2 AYU Detox Caps

7:00am: 8-12oz of room temperature water with a fresh squeeze of lemon or lime and a pinch of sea salt if desired

8:00am: Dr. Cabral Detox Shake #1

11:30am: Dr. Cabral Detox Shake #2

3:00pm: Dr. Cabral Detox Shake #3

6:30pm: Dr. Cabral Detox Shake #4

Get to bed as early as possible and conserve your energy

DAYS 3 - 7

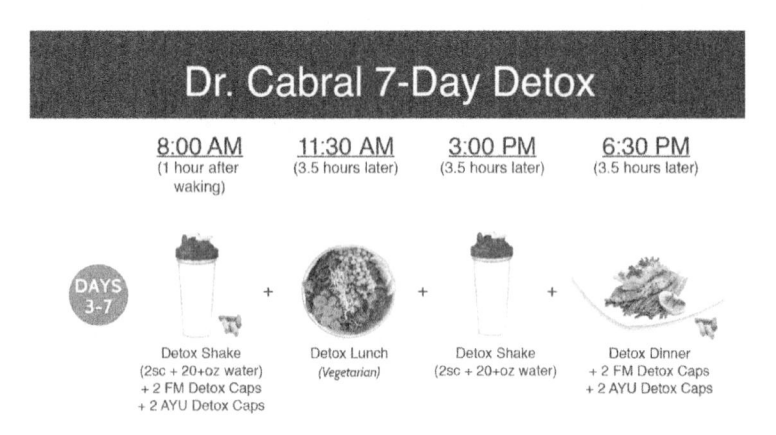

Dr. Cabral 7-Day Detox

DAYS 3-7

8:00 AM (1 hour after waking)
Detox Shake (2sc + 20+oz water) + 2 FM Detox Caps + 2 AYU Detox Caps

+

11:30 AM (3.5 hours later)
Detox Lunch *(Vegetarian)*

+

3:00 PM (3.5 hours later)
Detox Shake (2sc + 20+oz water)

+

6:30 PM (3.5 hours later)
Detox Dinner + 2 FM Detox Caps + 2 AYU Detox Caps

7:00am: 8-12oz of room temperature water with a fresh squeeze of lemon or lime and a pinch of sea salt if desired

8:00am: Dr. Cabral Detox Shake #1

11:30am: Vegan Lunch

3:00pm: Dr. Cabral Detox Shake #3

6:30pm: Vegan, Vegetarian or Paleo-style Dinner

DR. CABRAL DETOX HELPFUL TIPS

Remember, besides your daily 12-hour overnight fast, you're never going more than 3.5 hours without having a Dr. Cabral Detox shake or meal – This will leave you satiated all day long.

For the extended 14 & 21-Day Dr. Cabral Detox options, simply follow the 1st 7 day plan again as outlined above. However, just do the best you can and if you can't do a 2nd or 3rd set of 48 hours of shake fasting to begin each new week, you could just do 1 day, or simply following the days 3-7 detox meal plan for days 8-21. Either way, you'll still get great results and doing the detox in *any way you can* (especially the 1st time around) is so much better than not doing it at all!

If you're trying to decide on whether you should do the 7, 14, or 21-day Dr. Cabral Detox and you've never done a Functional Medicine detox protocol before I highly recommend completing the 21-day Dr. Cabral Detox (3 7 detoxes in a row) for maximum results. But of course, if you just want to dip your toes in the water and test it out 7-days would be great to start with as well and the results will still astound you!

Lastly, if you can't follow the exact times above as to when to have your shakes and meals, simply create your own schedule by spacing each meal and shake out approximately 3-4 hours. You should follow the plan as closely as you can, but you don't have to be perfect in order to get the benefits you're looking for. We've had firefighters, nurses, construction laborers, and dozens of other overnight and "off-hour" workers make their own schedule and still enjoy exceptional results.

Since I know you may have additional questions, simply go to *DrCabralDetox. com/faq* for all the most frequently asked questions and answers.

WHY YOU NEED SPECIFIC VITAMINS & NUTRITIONAL SUPPORT

Everyday you are being exposed to toxic chemicals in your food, water, clothing, plastics, bath & hair products, cosmetics, sunscreens, and even the air you breathe.

Unfortunately, there's just no escaping it…

But the good news is that you can keep up with eliminating these harmful chemicals by giving your body some additional support. As I mentioned before, food alone is no longer the sole answer, especially since much of it contains harmful pesticides (both "natural" and conventional) or has been grown in soil that is depleted of the nutrients your body needs.

Plus, as your body is breaking down its fat stores, additional toxins will be released from the fat. Did you know one of the reasons you may add body fat and can't seem to lose weight is because your adipose tissue (fat cells) are one of the safest places in your body to store away toxins when your body can't keep up with cleaning the blood?

That means when you're burning body fat and losing weight quickly, you'll want some additional support from the specific vitamins, antioxidants & amino acids that your liver needs to clean your body. Otherwise, you might pollute your blood with toxins, landing you back in the same toxic place you started.

Again, the whole process happens naturally since it's how your body is meant to work. We're just giving it a friendly boost – Which of course it is thankful for!

Please also note that you don't need to take the specific nutritional supplements I recommend forever – Just while you're on the detox and looking to maximize your results by following the proven Dr. Cabral Detox system.

Now I will show you exactly what supplements (and why) I recommend my private clients use in my practice and online. (You may purchase them anywhere you feel comfortable.)

WHAT YOU NEED FOR SPECIFIC VITAMINS & NUTRITIONAL SUPPORT

Now that you know that in order to *Empty Your Rain Barrel*™ and maximize your detox results you should be using specific vitamins, minerals, antioxidants & amino acids, I want to show you exactly what I recommend to my family, friends, and private clients. And of course, I personally use the Dr. Cabral Detox myself (4x a year seasonally).

It is no longer a mystery as to what your body needs in order to remove the harmful cancer causing chemicals. Earlier, I presented you with what nutrients your liver uses for both Phase 1 & 2 detoxification.

As a summary below, I have included which Functional Medicine nutritional supplements will help you best achieve that. Although there are many more you could take, the ones listed will give you the greatest amount of results per investment.

NUTRITIONAL SUPPLEMENT DETOX LIST

- **Activated Multi-Vitamin** (Phase 1 & 2 Detox Support)
- **Chelated Multi-Mineral** (Phase 1 & 2 Detox Support)
- **Electrolyte Formula** (Energy, Metabolism)
- **Methylated B-Complex** (Energy, Detox, Lower stress)
- **Pure Antioxidant Formula** (Detox, Anti-Aging)
- **Flax Seed** (Fiber, Detox, Omega-3, Improve bowel movements)
- **Psyllium Husk** (Fiber, Detox, Improve bowel movements)

- **Chromium** (Improves blood sugar stabilization)
- **Broccoli Extract** (Sulfurophane helps detox, kill cancer cells)
- **Liver Detox Co-factors** (Specific Phase 1 & 2 Detox Support)
- **l-Glutamine** (Detox, Tissue & Gut Repair, Muscle Sparing)
- **Vegan Protein** (Specific Amino Acids & Muscle Sparing)

(NOTE: Please keep in mind that if you choose to use the Dr. Cabral Detox 7, 14, or 21-day kit you get all of these nutritional supplements in just 3 bottles at a large savings. However, I'm also providing 3rd party products on my resource page so that you can make the best decision for you. Likewise, you may be able to find a local Functional Medicine doctor in your area that carries these specific products as well.)

DETOXING IS THE ANSWER

I honestly believe detoxification and cellular cleansing is the answer to what people are missing right now in order to transform their bodies and lives into something where they can wake up everyday and feel great. You simply must Empty Your Rain Barrel™ in order to get a fresh start.

The bottom line is this; I want the very best results for you. I honestly do care about your health and helping you overcome the wellness, weight loss, or aging issues you've been suffering from. Even if you've struggled in the past, I know *this will work for you*. If I could make just one recommendation it would be the Dr. Cabral Detox – It's the powerful and I've seen the real-world results in clinical practice to back it up…

HOW TO KEEP THE RESULTS COMING

I want to go one step further and that's to ensure you keep the results you got during your Dr. Cabral Detox coming.

To do this, I've designed a simple "Maintenance Plan" that I recommend using directly after the detox. It's literally what I've been using for years in my Boston Functional Medicine practice and it's the same exact meal plan I follow on a daily basis…

Just like the Dr. Cabral Detox, there are no elaborate meal plans or recipes to follow. I prefer you to enjoy the foods you like, while staying within the parameters of a healthy lifestyle and food selection.

HOW TO MAINTAIN YOUR RESULTS

The first question I'm typically asked is, *"can I can ever go back to 'normal' eating…"*

My answer is always, *"how would you define normal?"*

If you're asking if you can eat pizza, and pasta, sandwiches and pastries on a daily basis my answer would be that I can't recommend that, since those foods do not align with your goals of being healthy, happy, and living a better quality life.

However, I am a firm believer that once you've done a 21-Day Dr. Cabral Detox or you're feeling well again, that you absolutely can have one cheat meal per week. This is literally one meal per week where you can eat those foods that you crave and do not want to remove from your life forever. I typically do the same thing once per week and usually enjoy a nice bowl of pasta (and bread!) or a dessert.

Some people can increase this to 2 cheat meals per week (at least 48 hours apart), but that is dictated solely by if they start to slide back in terms of health or weight gain. I'll leave that decision up to you, but my advice would be to simply start at one cheat per week for the first month.

MY HIGHEST RECOMMENDATION

If there is one recommendation I can make that will help you more than anything else in terms of maintaining your results, it's to keep your breakfast easy to digest and high in water content.

This will allow you to not give away your energy first thing in the morning towards digesting heavy fatty foods like bacon or sausage. Instead, you'll be focused on low glycemic, high fiber, high antioxidant fruit like berries.

My highest recommendation, and the same one that finally gave me back the energy I was seeking, is to start your day with a fruit smoothie. It's so simple, inexpensive and easy to do that there's really no equal alternative. To remind you, smoothies free up your digestive energy, the energy you'd exhaust digesting fibrous, fatty, or protein-dense foods.

(Note: To download my free smoothie guide for after your detox simply go to: http://stephencabral.com/270-2/ (There is also a free podcast on my favorite smoothies), or StephenCabral.com/rbe)

Making a smoothie is literally as easy as pouring 8oz of water, 8oz of unsweetened vanilla nut milk, 1 cup of frozen blueberries, and adding 2 scoops of your Daily Nutritional Support powder, which is your full activated multivitamin, mineral, antioxidant, daily detox support, and 15g of vegan protein powder into a blender.

You can add plenty of more ingredients, but if you do nothing else, this is my highest recommendation. Again, most people don't have the time to make an elaborate healthy breakfast and so a morning smoothie is truly the best option to keep your results coming!

Now let's make this even easier and give you a sample daily meal plan as to how my private wellness clients and I maintain our results:

SAMPLE DAILY MAINTENANCE PLAN
BREAKFAST

- Fruit Smoothie with Daily Nutritional Support powder. See my "Purple Crush" smoothie recipe in the resource section in the back of this book or at StephenCabral.com/rbe
- You may add a bowl of gluten-free oatmeal, buckwheat, or granola on the side if you're looking to keep your weight up

LUNCH

- 2+ cups of vegetables
- 1/2-1 cup of gluten free starch (yams, sweet potatoes, yucca, etc.) or gluten free grain (rice, quinoa, buckwheat, oats, etc.)
- 1/2-1c of protein
- 1-2 TBSP of healthy fat
- Season to taste (sea salt, herbs, etc.)

MID-AFTERNOON SNACK (OPTIONAL)

- ¼- ½ cup of nuts
- or, Cut of vegetables or rice crackers and 2-3 TBSP of hummus or guacamole
- or, 1 cup of berries or fruit
- or, Fresh pressed vegetable juice
- or, 2nd smoothie

DINNER

- 2+ cups of vegetables
- 1/2-1 cup of gluten free starch (yams, sweet potatoes, yucca, etc.) or gluten free grain (rice, quinoa, buckwheat, oats, etc.)
- 1/2-1c of protein
- 1-2 TBSP of healthy fat
- Season to taste (sea salt, herbs, etc.)

Only consume starch at dinner if looking to maintain your current weight or gain weight.

If you're thinking to yourself that this resembles the Dr. Cabral Detox days 3-7 you would be correct! The additional items that have been added back in are fruit 1-2x/day and gluten-free starches like sweet potatoes, yams, yucca, oats, rice, quinoa, etc. The serving sizes are just suggestions and you can adjust them as needed based on your weight and energy requirements.

Remember, the secret to staying healthy is to not get sick again in the first place! This is why I've designed the maintenance plan to be a very simple daily clean eating plan with a 1-2 time a week cheat meal to still enjoy some of your favorite foods...

IT'S TIME TO GET STARTED

Many years ago, I was where you are right now...

I was frustrated with starting and stopping, trying and failing, and just not knowing what I should do in order to get my body back to a state of balance. I understand where you are and what you're going through.

My goal with the *Rain Barrel Effect* was to simply show you, how you got here, and what you need to do next in order to get well.

The truth is that adding more to your body is not always the answer. Often times, the reason we've failed in the past, is because what we really needed to do is take something away – Not put more into it. You simply must get rid of years of toxic and inflammatory build up.

I can honestly tell you that after 250,000 client appointments and seeing daily unsolicited success stories come pouring in from Dr. Cabral Detox users, that the Dr. Cabral Detox and *Emptying Your Rain Barrel*™ is the answer you've been searching for. It has worked for me, my private clients, and thousands of others just like you.

I also want you to know that it does not matter to me if you use my clinically proven Dr. Cabral Detox or just purchase all of the vitamins, minerals, antioxidants, and amino acids separately. I want you to do what you feel is best for you, but most of all I want you to finally get well, lose the weight, and feel alive again!

Right now, I'm probably as excited as you are (if not more) for you to join our community and experience the power and results of the Dr. Cabral Detox. I truly wish you the best of success, and I can't wait to hear your success story soon!

To get create your own success story and get started today, go to DrCabralDetox.com or this book's resource page for details: StephenCabral.com/rbe

The Best Time To Start

As the old proverb goes, "The best time to start was yesterday. The second best time is today."

We covered a lot of material in this book. I'm sure some of it you have heard before, but maybe not in this context. Or, perhaps this was the very first time you saw how the entire puzzle comes together and makes sense.

Regardless, you now know everything you need to get started. You do not need to be perfect or even get it all right in order to start.

Too many of us, myself included, often do less than we are capable of simply because we have the faulty belief that we always need more data before taking that first step. This is a mistake. To be honest, there is no way you can ever collect enough data or knowledge to know every pitfall or obstacle you may encounter and how to prepare for it.

The truth is that you'll only get those answers once you begin on your quest. You must begin to walk down the path before knowing what the next step will be. The most successful people follow this rule and my hope is you model that same success habit.

SUCCESS LEAVES CLUES

Doing your best really is good enough. Never compare yourself to anyone else – for better or worse. Simply, follow the DESTRESS Protocol™ outlined in this book.

Everyday, take just one more step forward.

This is literally how I got well. I gathered more knowledge and then implemented it. I found out what worked and what didn't. I then recalibrated each time and learned from both my mistakes and wins. I brushed my mistakes aside and tried to build off my wins. I learned by trial and error. Until I met my mentor, I learned the hard way, but eventually I made it anyway…

The good news is that you don't need to learn the hard way like I did. I made all the mistakes so that you don't have to. Let my pain, struggle, and eventual success motivate you to achieve your own great results, but do not repeat my failures.

HEALTHY PEOPLE CAN'T BE SICK

I have truly laid out the exact plan of how to renew and rejuvenate your body at the deepest level possible.

This is where all underlying root causes lie – that's why when you rebalance these areas included in the DESTRESS Protocol™ you will Empty Your Rain Barrel™ and become whole again. Sickness, disease, weight gain, fatigue, skin issues, low mood, headaches, etc. cannot live in your new healthy body.

The great thing is that when you finally Empty Your Rain Barrel™, you are going to begin to experience feelings you may not have felt for years – if ever. We've had so many people write in letting us know they never knew they could enjoy so much *energy*, so much *joy*, so much *blissfulness*, and renewed *vitality* by letting go of internal and external toxins in their life.

Please also keep in mind that most of the healing protocols outlined in this book are free or merely substitutions for things you're already using or doing now. Do not let lifestyle or financial constraints hold you back from what you can do. Little by little, begin to make changes that feel right to you. Begin with just one action and go from there.

As stated before, you'll get the most noticeable results by completing the 7, 14, or 21-day Dr. Cabral Detox, or a comparable protocol. Let these results be the catalyst that propels you forward to attaining even greater accomplishments in your life. Let changing your body be the springboard to changing your life!

"EACH ONE, TEACH ONE."

One of the main reasons I went into Naturopathic and Functional Medicine was to help people take back control of their body, so that they can have the health, energy, and confidence to do and be more in their life. Without your health, it's difficult to accomplish everything else you want and dream of.

I believe in you and the potential that you have inside. I also want you to optimize your health, body, and overall vitality, so that you can be a role model for your family, friends, and co-workers.

I want your success and enthusiasm for improving your overall life to be so contagious that others can't help but to ask you what you've been doing! This will allow you to share with them how you've made simple lifestyle changes that when added together have created a whole that is so much more powerful than any one of its individual parts.

You will then be able to pay it forward and be the go-to health person in your group that can guide one more person to a healthier life. A person that without you may have never made their own change.

CREATE YOUR OWN HAPPY ENDING

In the opening chapter of this book I shared with you the troubled story of Sara's struggle with bloating, fatigue, low mood, anxiety, weight gain, decreased libido, and skin issues amongst others...

She wasn't happy and that spread through her entire life – Into her relationships, job, and with over eating. When we first met, she still had all the same issues, but one thing had changed – *She was now ready to change.* She had opened her mind to the possibility of creating a new healthy life in both mind and body.

I let her know that she was not alone – She was now a part of a community that understood her. I also let her know that since we've all been where she was, we could help guide her out of these troubled times. So, the first thing Sara did was simply begin to believe she could achieve better health and her ideal body. After renewed hope, she then went about implementing the DESTRESS Protocol™.

I also instructed Sara to complete the 21-Day Dr. Cabral Detox before our next follow up visit. 3 weeks went by without me hearing a word from her, but during our next appointment I could immediately see something was different...

Sara walked into my office with a new vibrant glow I had now come to recognize. As she sat down across from me with tears in her eyes and barely being able to contain the smile she had been trying to hold back, that's when we both broke down laughing knowing she had made the breakthrough she had been searching for – *She was now a new person.*

Although she still had some improvements to make and she wasn't perfect, she was now well on her way to becoming the person she'd always dreamed of. Her skin had cleared up, her sleep improved, her anxiety diminished, her energy and libido increased, and she had no more bloating. But best of all, she told me she could finally be herself in her relationship again.

Just writing this and recounting Sara's story makes me emotional. This is why I do what I do and I want this for everyone and that includes *you*.

THE TIME IS NOW

I know how busy everyone is. After seeing more than 250,000 client appointments in my practice, my team and I understand that there is never going to be a perfect time to get started. This is why you must start now. In one week, your motivation will start to dip and you'll have more obligations.

This is life.

The only remedy to this is action. And the only way to not look back weeks, months, or years from now with regret from not starting sooner is to get started today. Like the old me, the issues you're facing will most likely not go away on their own. They need some type of transformative action. They need you to start by taking that first step.

Begin by completing your own 21-day detox, while trying to implement just 1 improvement from each of the "Diet, Exercise, Stress, Toxin, Rest, Emotion, Supplements, and Success" categories. Choose an easy one. Then build off of that win. Then add another. This is how success is built.

It's not fancy, but it is effective.

After this final chapter, I've included a resource section with what I believe to be the most useful links to implement the DESTRESS Protocol™. These same resources, plus dozens more updated ones are available at StephenCabral.com/rbe

Although I never want to repeat the hard times I had to go through many years ago, I'm envious of you beginning your journey. You have so much to look forward to. I know it can feel impossible, overwhelming, or too high of a mountain to climb, but that is how everyone feels before starting anything new for the first time.

I can't wait to hear your success story about how much healthier, happier, and more vibrant you feel! It won't be long and when it happens, I do hope you'll write in and share your success with me. Seeing your success story and feeling your joy continues to propel me to do more.

Thank you for coming along on this journey with me, and I do hope I was able to instill in you the knowledge that you can and will get well, lose the weight, and finally feel alive again!

Now it's time for *you* to Empty Your Rain Barrel™!

Ayubowan,

Dr. Stephen Cabral
Doctor of Naturopathy
Ayurvedic & Functional Medicine Practitioner

About the Author

At 17-years old, Stephen Cabral became extremely sick and was shuffled around from doctor to doctor looking for some type of diagnosis of why he suffered the way he did.

After being told it was all in his head and then later being given multiple diagnosis's of "dis-ease" states that he would need to medicate and manage for the rest of his life, he sought out alternative treatments. It was in these meetings with Naturopathic, Ayurvedic, and Functional Medicine Doctors that he was given hope for the first time.

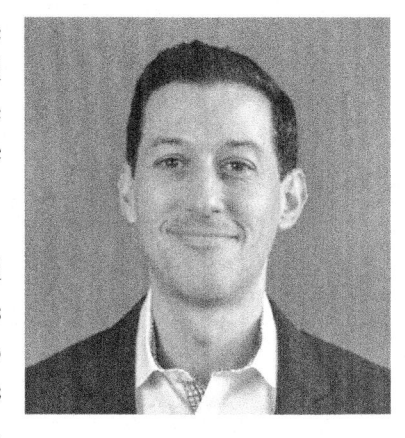

Stephen went on to read thousands of books in his quest to discover the "missing piece to the puzzle." His own mentor in health recommended he go back to school to get his Doctorate of Naturopathy. Dr. Cabral did exactly that, but he was not yet satisfied with his education, so he went overseas to uncover the answers he was looking for.

It was through studying and interning at clinics in India, Sri Lanka, China, Europe, and all over the US, that he finally found what he was searching for. It was the lost information on detoxifying and rejuvenating the body that Dr. Cabral re-discovered and turned into a new system of medicine that combines the best of ancient wisdom with state-of-the-art Functional Medicine. His mission is to share the message of hope and healing to those that need it the most.

Dr. Cabral practices in Boston, MA where he also lives with his wife, 2 young daughters, and their crazy French bulldog, Moose.

RBE Success Resources & Recommendations

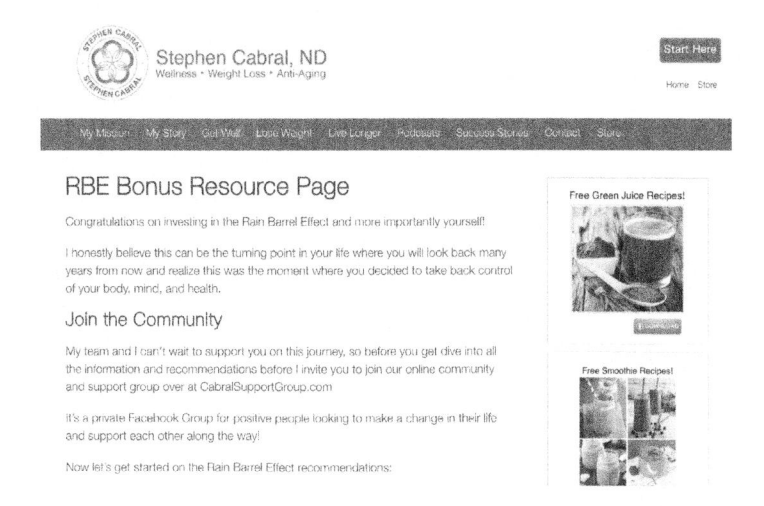

I know I mentioned this resource page many times throughout the book, but that was done on purpose. My goal is to make sure that you never stop learning, growing, and fueling your passion for all things wellness, weight loss, and anti-aging. Therefore, in order to do that you must stay up-to-date with the latest recommendations and resources.

Research and products get upgraded with time, but the one constant is the truth. As a result, you'll only find recommendations that I personally use or recommend to my family, friends, and those I care for in my private practice. I don't compromise on health and well-being and I want to make sure you don't have to either. The follow pages contain our RBE community's favorite links!

THE RAIN BARREL EFFECT (RBE) RESOURCE PAGE

All the *updated* RBE recommendations, workouts, diet plans, recipes, labs, detox systems, home products, and so much are contained on this private web page for book readers only!

- **StephenCabral.com/rbe**

DR. CABRAL'S PERSONAL RECOMMENDATIONS

All of Dr. Cabral's at-home lab testing, daily supplement recommendations, specialty supplements, and other items he uses in his Boston and International Concierge practice are at:

- **StephenCabral.com/store**

DR. CABRAL DETOX

Dr. Cabral's most popular solution to the health & body issues that ail you. Join the community and the thousands of others that are getting amazing results everyday using the 7, 14, or 21-day Dr. Cabral Detox. You can find details at:

- **DrCabralDetox.com**

DR. CABRAL DAILY PROTOCOL

After you finish your Dr. Cabral Detox this is what Dr. Cabral (and his family) personally uses each morning and recommends in his practice in order to get every vitamin, mineral, electrolyte, protein, and antioxidant you need to start your day. Plus, you get the whole food nutrition of 22 organic fruits & vegetables and 50 billion dairy-free probiotics to help your gut. Details available at:

- **StephenCabral.com/daily-protocol**

TOP 7 WELLNESS & WEIGHT LOSS SMOOTHIES

One of the most healing regimens you can begin is including a daily smoothie for breakfast and/or as a mid-afternoon snack. The easy to digest nutrition will literally change your life. The link below contains the most popular wellness & weight loss smoothies as voted on by the Cabral Community. It also includes Dr. Cabral's personal favorite "Purple Crush Smoothie!"

- **StephenCabral.com/smoothie-recipes**

8 ENERGY, IMMUNITY & DIGESTIVE GREENS DRINK RECIPES

We urge you to take the "Cabral Green's Drink Challenge" and try adding in the Superfood power of 22 organic fruits & vegetables into your life. You'll never look, feel, or be the same again! These 8 "favorites" are recipes created to make your *Daily Fruit & Vegetable Blend* powder even more enjoyable!

- **StephenCabral.com/greens-drink-recipes**

Resources

INTRODUCTION

[1] National Toxicology Program. About NTP. https://ntp.niehs.nih.gov/about/index.html

[2] H. Whiteman. 1 in 2 people will develop cancer in their lifetime. *Medical News Today.* http://www.medicalnewstoday.com/articles/288916.php

[3] AARDA. Autoimmune disease statistics. https://www.aarda.org/news-information/statistics/

[4] CDC. Heart disease facts and statistics. https://www.cdc.gov/heartdisease/facts.htm

[5] CDC. High blood pressure facts. https://www.cdc.gov/bloodpressure/facts.htm

[6] Migraine.com. Migraine statistics. https://migraine.com/migraine-statistics/

[7] ADAA. Facts and statistics. https://adaa.org/about-adaa/press-room/facts-statistics

[8] NIH: NIDDK. Overweight and obesity statistics. https://www.niddk.nih.gov/health-information/health-statistics/overweight-obesity

[9] Belluck, P. (2005). Children's life expectancy being cut short by obesity. http://www.nytimes.com/2005/03/17/health/childrens-life-expectancy-being-cut-short-by-obesity.html

CHAPTER 1

[1] ARDA. Autoimmune disease statistics. https://www.aarda.org/news-information/statistics/

[2] Alzheimer's Association. Alzheimer's disease: Statistics. http://www.alzheimers-illinois.org/statistics.pdf

[3] American Cancer Society. Lifetime risk of developing or dying from cancer. https://www.cancer.org/cancer/cancer-basics/lifetime-probability-of-developing-or-dying-from-cancer.html

[4] CDC. Diabetes. https://www.cdc.gov/diabetes/pdfs/library/diabetesreportcard2014.pdf

[5] CDC. Heart disease facts and statistics. https://www.cdc.gov/heartdisease/facts.htm

[6] CDC. Arthritis related statistics. https://www.cdc.gov/arthritis/data_statistics/arthritis-related-stats.htm

[7] Christopher, J. L. et. al. (2010). Ranking 37th — Measuring the performance of the U.S. health care system. *The New England Journal of Medicine*. 362: 98-99. http://www.nejm.org/doi/full/10.1056/NEJMp0910064#t=article

[8] Gray, L. (2014). Will today's children die younger than their parents? *BBC News*. http://www.bbc.com/news/magazine-28191865

[9] CDC. Autism spectrum disorder. https://www.cdc.gov/ncbddd/autism/data.html

[10] EWG. Children, health risks, and autism spectrum disorder. http://www.ewg.org/kid-safe-chemicals-act-blog/ewg-research/

[11] EWG. Body burden: The pollutants in newborns. http://www.ewg.org/research/body-burden-pollution-newborns#.WYzkzcaZO9Y

[12] Anand, P. et. al. Cancer is a Preventable Disease that Requires Major Lifestyle Changes. *Pharmaceutical Research, 25*(9): 2097–2116 https://www.ncbi.nlm.nih.gov/pmc/articles/PMC2515569/

[13] Campbell, A. (2014). Autoimmunity and the gut. *Autoimmune Disease.* 2014: 152428. https://www.ncbi.nlm.nih.gov/pmc/articles/PMC4036413/

[14] Palmer, R. F. (2006). Environmental mercury release, special education rates, and autism disorder: an ecological study of Texas. *Health and Place. 12*(2): 203-209. https://www.ncbi.nlm.nih.gov/pubmed/16338635

[15] Goyer, R. A. and G. Cherian. (2011). *Toxicology of Metals: Biochemical Aspect,* Springer Press.

[16] ASTDR. Cadmium Toxicity. https://www.atsdr.cdc.gov/csem.asp?=6&po=12

[17] Miller, et al. (2002). Mechanisms of action of arsenic trioxide. *Cancer Research, 62*(14):3893-903. https://www.ncbi.nlm.nih.gov/pubmed/12124315

[18] Smith, J. Genetically Modified Soy Linked to Sterility, Infant Mortality in Hamsters, HuffPost. http://www.huffingtonpost.com/jeffrey-smith/genetically-modified-soy_b_544575.html

[19] Savvani, A, et. al. (2013) IGF-IEc expression is associated with advanced clinical and pathological stage of prostate cancer. *Anticancer Re*search, *33*(6): 2441-5. https://www.researchgate.net/publication/237092550_IGF-

[20] Green Living. *The Dangers of Preservatives.* http://greenliving.lovetoknow.com/dangers-food-additives-preservatives

[21] USRTK. Aspartame: Decades of science point to serious health risks. https://usrtk.org/sweeteners/aspartame_health_risks/

[22] Center for Science of Public Interest. CSPI Downgrades Sucralose from "Caution" to "Avoid. https://cspinet.org/new/201602081.html

[23] Consumer Safety Watch. Roundup weed killer. https://www.consumer-safetywatch.com/lawsuit/roundup-weed-killer

[24] Sustainable Baby Steps. *The dangers of pesticides.* http://www.sustainable-babysteps.com/dangers-of-pesticides.html

[25] The DDT Story. http://www.panna.org/resources/ddt-story

[26] Blair, A. (1982). *Cancer risks associated with agriculture: epidemiologic evidence.* Basic Life Science, 21:93-111. https://www.ncbi.nlm.nih.gov/pubmed/7150208

[27] WHO. Pesticides. http://www.who.int/ceh/capacity/Pesticides.pdf

[28] Benzinga. (2017). New study links glycosaphate with autism. https://www.benzinga.com/pressreleases/17/03/r9140572/new-study-links-weed-killer-glyphosate-with-autism

[29] Reader's Digest. *The dark side of the perfectly manicured American lawn.* http://www.rd.com/home/gardening/lawn-fertilizer-dangers/

[30] Fluroide Alert.org. (2012). http://fluoridealert.org/studies/caries01/

[31] Sparrowdancer, M. (2011). *Fluoride poisoning: It's all over.* http://rense.com/general93/fluo.htm

[32] NT. (2016). Harvard researchers link fluoridated water to ADHD, autism and other childhood mental health disorders. http://

newstarget.com/2016-01-26-harvard-researchers-link-fluoridated-water-to-adhd-autism-and-other-childhood-mental-health-disorers.html

[33] Group, Dr. Edward. (2015). *Shocking dangers of fluoride.* http://www.globalhealingcenter.com/natural-health/9-shocking-dangers-of-fluoride/

[34] Harvard Health Publications. (2011). *Drugs in the water.* https://www.health.harvard.edu/newsletter_article/drugs-in-the-water

[35] State of the Planet. (201). *From wastewater to drinking water.* http://blogs.ei.columbia.edu/2011/04/04/from-wastewater-to-drinking-water/

[36] WHO. Electromagnetic Hypersensitivity. http://www.who.int/peh-emf/publications/facts/fs296/en/

[37] National Cancer Institute: *Magnetic Field Exposure and Cancer: Questions and Answers.* http://www.cancer.gov/cancertopics/factsheet/risk/magnetic-fields

[38] World Health Organization: *What Are Electromagnetic Fields?* http://www.who.int/peh-emf/about/WhatisEMF/en/

[39] NIH. *Cell phones and cancer risk.* https://www.cancer.gov/about-cancer/causes-prevention/risk/radiation/cell-phones-fact-sheet

[40] ibid

[41] Daily Mail. *How the air in your house is making you ill.* http://www.dailymail.co.uk/health/article-2920391/How-AIR-house-making-ill-drying-washing-using-gas-cooker-15-million-homes-affected-Toxic-Home-Syndrome-increases-risk-heart-disease-cancer.html

[42] EWG. *The trouble with ingredients in sunscreens.* http://www.ewg.org/sunscreen/report/the-trouble-with-sunscreen-chemicals/#.WYzdlMaZO9Y

[43] EWG. CDC: Americans carry body burden of toxic sunscreen chemical. http://www.ewg.org/news/testimony-official-correspondence/cdc-americans-carry-body-burden-toxic-sunscreen-chemical#.WYzcV8aZO9Y

[44] Mayo Clinic News Network. (2013). *7 in 10 Americans take prescription drugs.* http://newsnetwork.mayoclinic.org/discussion/nearly-7-in-10-americans-take-prescription-drugs-mayo-clinic-olmsted-medical-center-find/

[45] Mayo Clinic. *Statin side effects: Weigh the benefits and the risks.* http://www.mayoclinic.org/diseases-conditions/high-blood-cholesterol/in-depth/statin-side-effects/art-20046013

[46] Mercola: *The truth about statin drugs revealed.* http://articles.mercola.com/sites/articles/archive/2010/07/20/the-truth-about-statin-drugs-revealed.aspx

[47] Everyday Health. *What is Prilosec?* https://www.everydayhealth.com/drugs/prilosec

[48] J. Tamney. (2010). Healthcare 16% of GDP https://www.forbes.com/2010/01/31/health-care-gdp-reform-opinions-columnists-john-tamny.html

[49] CDC. Parasites. https://www.cdc.gov/parasites/index.html

CHAPTER 2

[1] Duncan, D. (2006). The pollution within. National Geographic. http://www2.onu.edu/~b-boulanger/CE3231PollutionWithin.pdf

[2] CDC. CDC estimates 1 in 68 children has been identified with autism spectrum disorder. https://www.cdc.gov/media/releases/2014/p0327-autism-spectrum-disorder.html

CHAPTER 3

[1] Ramaswamy, S. The benefits of Ayurveda self-Massage "Abhyanga" http://www.chopra.com/articles/the-benefits-of-ayurveda-self-massage

[2] Bhatted, S. (2011). A study on Vasantika Vamana (therapeutic emesis in spring season: *A preventive measure for diseases of Kapha origin*. *Āyurvedāloka*, 32(2): 181–186. https://www.ncbi.nlm.nih.gov/pmc/articles/PMC3296337/

[3] Sisson, M. Infrared Sauna Roundup. http://www.marksdailyapple.com/dear-mark-infrared-sauna-roundup/

[4] Herron, R.E, and J. B. Fagan. (2002). Lipophil-mediated reduction of toxicants in humans: an evaluation of an ayurvedic detoxification procedure. *Alternative Therapeutic Health and Medicine*. 8(5):40-51. https://www.ncbi.nlm.nih.gov/pubmed/12233802

[5] Jiang, L (2012). Alexis Carrel's Immortal Chick Heart Tissue Cultures (1912-1946). https://embryo.asu.edu/pages/alexis-carrels-immortal-chick-heart-tissue-cultures-1912-1946

CHAPTER 4

[1] Sustainable table. Antibiotics. http://www.sustainabletable.org/257/antibiotics

[2] Axe, J. The dangers of farmed fish. https://draxe.com/the-dangers-of-farmed-fish/

[3] BottomLine. How your APOe gene can lead to diabetes or heart disease http://bottomlineinc.com/health/prevention/how-your-apoe-genes-lead-to-diabetes-or-heart-disease

[4] Christensen A. S. et. al. (2013). Effect of fruit restriction on glycemic control in patients with type 2 diabetes--a randomized trial. *Nutritional Journal.* 12:29. doi: 10.1186/1475-2891-12-29. https://www.ncbi.nlm.nih.gov/pubmed/23497350

[5] Scott.Net. A heart surgeon speaks out about what really causes heart disease. https://www.sott.net/article/242516-Heart-surgeon-speaks-out-on-what-really-causes-heart-disease

CHAPTER 5

[1] Sustainable table. Antibiotics. http://www.sustainabletable.org/257/antibiotics

[2] Axe, J. The dangers of farmed fish. https://draxe.com/the-dangers-of-farmed-fish/

[3] BottomLine. How your APOe gene can lead to diabetes or heart disease http://bottomlineinc.com/health/prevention/how-your-apoe-genes-lead-to-diabetes-or-heart-disease

[4] Christensen A. S. et. al. (2013). Effect of fruit restriction on glycemic control in patients with type 2 diabetes--a randomized trial. *Nutritional Journal.* 12:29. doi: 10.1186/1475-2891-12-29. https://www.ncbi.nlm.nih.gov/pubmed/23497350

CHAPTER 7

[1] CDC. Fourth national report on human exposure to environmental toxins. https://www.cdc.gov/biomonitoring/pdf/fourthreport_updatedtables_feb2015.pdf

[2] United States House of Representatives report, 1989.

[3] CBS News. Report: Cancer Causing Chemical Found In 90 Percent of America's Water Systems http://philadelphia.cbslocal.com/2016/09/21/report-cancer-causing-chemical-found-in-90-percent-of-americas-water-systems/

[4] SmartKlean Blog. The Top 12 Cancer-Causing products in the Average Home https://smartklean.wordpress.com/2011/02/23/the-top-12-cancer-causing-products-in-the-average-home/

[5] Environmental Alternatives. Facts and statistics about toxins. http://www.enviroalternatives.com/nontoxichome.html

[6] Black, T. 7 toxins lurking in your deodorant. https://dontmesswithmama.com/7-toxins-lurking-in-your-deodorant/

[7] Mercola. (2015). Toxic Toothpaste Ingredients You Need to Avoid http://articles.mercola.com/sites/articles/archive/2015/09/09/toxic-toothpaste-ingredients.aspx

[8] Forbes. The most toxic toys. https://www.forbes.com/2008/12/16/toys-product-safety-biz-commerce-cx_wp_1216toxictoys.html

[9] Weston A. Price. Nutrition, fluoridation, and dental health. https://www.westonaprice.org/health-topics/dentistry/nutrition-fluoridation-and-dental-health/

[10] Hodges, R. E. (2015). Modulation of Metabolic Detoxification Pathways Using Foods and Food-Derived Components: A Scientific Review with Clinical Application. *Journal of Nutritional Metabolism.* https://www.ncbi.nlm.nih.gov/pmc/articles/PMC4488002/

[11] SelfHacked. 19 Incredible Science-Based Health Benefits of Regular Sauna Use https://selfhacked.com/2016/05/08/reasons-sweating-far-often/#2_Saunas_Increase_Longevity

[12] The Infared Sauna Effect. http://www.the-infrared-sauna-effect.com/introduction-to-the-sauna.html

[13] Dr. Mercola. 17 Micrograms of lead in your body lowers your iq by 10 points http://articles.mercola.com/sites/articles/archive/2012/03/21/dr-clement-on-detoxification.aspx

[14] Dr. Lawrence Wilson. Coffee enemas, http://www.drlwilson.com/articles/COFFEE%20ENEMA.HTM

[15] Hyman, Mark. (2011). Glutathione: The mother of all antioxidants. http://www.huffingtonpost.com/dr-mark-hyman/glutathione-the-mother-of_b_530494.html

CHAPTER 8

[1] The Sympathetic and Parasympathetic Nervous Systems. http://study.com/academy/lesson/the-sympathetic-and-parasympathetic-nervous-systems.html

[2] Chan, S. and M. Debono. (2010). Replication of cortisol circadian rhythm: New Advances in hydrocortisone replacement therapy. Therapeutic advances in Endocrinology and Metabolism, 1(3): 129-138. https://www.ncbi.nlm.nih.gov/pmc/articles/PMC3475279/

[3] Akerstedt, T. (2009). Sleep Loss and Fatigue in Shift Work and Shift Work Disorder. *Sleep Medicine Clinic, 4*(2): 257-271. https://www.ncbi.nlm.nih.gov/pmc/articles/PMC2904525/

[4] Lucas, R. (2014). Measuring and using light in the melanopsin age. *Trends in Neuroscience, 37*(1): 1-9. https://www.ncbi.nlm.nih.gov/pmc/articles/PMC4699304/

[5] Applied Neurotechnologies. The effects of TV on your brain. http://appliedneurotec.com/neuroscience/effects-of-tv-on-your-brain/

CHAPTER 9

[1] Brian L. Weiss. (2012). *Many Lives, Many Masters. Simon & Schuster.* https://www.amazon.com/dp/B007EDYNAO/ref=dp-kindle-redirect?_encoding=UTF8&btkr=1

[2] Yano, J. (2015). Indigenous Bacteria from the Gut Microbiota Regulate Host Serotonin Biosynthesis. *Cell, 161*(2():, 264-276 http://www.cell.com/cell/abstract/S0092-8674(15)00248-2?_returnURL=http://linkinghub.elsevier.com/retrieve/pii/S0092867415002482?showall=true

[3] Khalsa, D. S. (2015). Stress, Meditation, and Alzheimer's Disease Prevention: Where The Evidence Stands. *Journal of Alzheimer's Disease, 48*(1): 1-12. https://www.ncbi.nlm.nih.gov/pmc/articles/PMC4923750/

[4] Dr. David Perlmutter. Gut inflammation and the brain. http://www.drperlmutter.com/gut-inflammation-affects-brain/

[5] Simopoulos, A. P. (2002). The importance of the ratio of omega-6/omega-3 essential fatty acids. *Biomedical Pharmacotherapy*, 56(8):365-79. https://www.ncbi.nlm.nih.gov/pubmed/12442909

CHAPTER 10

[1] Berardi, J., Ph.D.Chances are you've got a deficiency. https://www.precisionnutrition.com/balanced-diet-isnt-enough

[2] CDC. Childhood obesity facts. (2014). http://www.cdc.gov/healthyyouth/obesity/facts.htm

[3] Kreb-Smith S, et. al. (2010). Americans do not meet federal dietary recommendations. *Journal of Nutrition*, *140*(10):1832-1838. https://www.ncbi.nlm.nih.gov/pmc/articles/PMC2937576/

[4] NPR. (2016). Is organic more nutritious? New study adds to the evidence. *The Salt.* http://www.npr.org/sections/thesalt/2016/02/18/467136329/is-organic-more-nutritious-new-study-adds-to-the-evidence

[5] Davis, D. (2004). Changes in USDA food composition data for 43 garden crops, 1950 to 1999. *Journal of the American College of Nutrition*, *23*(6):669-82. https://www.ncbi.nlm.nih.gov/pubmed/15637215

[6] Lee, S. et. al. Preharvest and postharvest factors influencing vitamin C content of horticultural crops, *Postharvest Biology and Technology, 20*(3): 207-220. https://doi.org/10.1016/S0925-5214(00)00133-2

[7] EPA. Nutrient Pollution. https://www.epa.gov/nutrientpollution/problem

[8] OSU. (2008). Here's the scoop on chemical and organic fertilizers. http://extension.oregonstate.edu/gardening/node/955

[9] Mahoney, C. R. et. al. (2005). Effect of breakfast composition on cognitive processes in elementary school children. *Physiological Behavior. 85*(5):635-645. https://www.ncbi.nlm.nih.gov/pubmed/16085130

[10] Herrero, *L. et. al.* (2006). A study on breakfast and school performance in a group of adolescents. *Nutrition and Hospitality. 21*(3):346-352. https://www.ncbi.nlm.nih.gov/pubmed/16771116

[11] CNN. (2017). Thousands of skittles end up on an icy road. http://www.cnn.com/2017/01/19/health/spilled-skittles-road-trnd/index.html

[12] Sustainable table. Antibiotics http://www.sustainabletable.org/257/antibiotics

[13] Farmed salmon: The most toxic food in the world. http://www.justnaturallife.com/farmed-salmon-one-of-the-most-toxic-foods-in-the-world/

[14] Natural News. Conventional chicken fed arsenic. http://www.naturalnews.com/042679_conventional_chicken_arsenic_fda.html

[15] Harvard T. Chan. Do vitamins make you healthier. https://www.health.harvard.edu/mens-health/do-multivitamins-make-you-healthier

[16] FullScript. Most prescribed supplements. https://fullscript.com/blog/most-prescribed-supplements-july-2017

[17] ibid.

[18] Josh Axe. 4 steps to heal leaky gut and autoimmune disease. https://draxe.com/4-steps-to-heal-leaky-gut-and-autoimmune-disease/

CHAPTER 11

[1] Campbell, A. (2014). Autoimmunity and the gut. *Autoimmune diseases.* doi: 10.1155/2014/152428 https://www.ncbi.nlm.nih.gov/pmc/articles/PMC4036413/

[2] Axe, J. How to reverse diabetes naturally in 30 days or less. https://draxe.com/how-to-reverse-diabetes-naturally-in-30-days-or-less/

Printed in Great Britain
by Amazon